OPEN THIS BOOK AND SAY "AHHH!"

"Personally knowing Dr. Sadler's excellent clinical skills, it's a delight to see how an accomplished physician can translate quality health information into readable, enjoyable bites that anyone will enjoy and absorb. This book is an outstanding contribution to digestible understanding of health and disease. By combining factual information, good writing skills, humility, and wit, she has honed a niche that readers will quickly enjoy. Sound tips for health and health maintenance are interspersed with humorous anecdotes. I am looking forward to volume 2."

– Carl E. Couch, MD, MMM
  VP Innovation
  Baylor Scott & White Health, Dallas
  Author, *Accountable*

"Dr. Jane Sadler is one of the most compassionate physicians I have ever met. I'm always overwhelmed by her amazing attention to detail in caring for her patients. And, Dr. Sadler's newspaper columns and blog are superb! I highly recommend!"

– Patty Granville, Producer, Garland Summer Musicals

"I find the topics of Dr. Jane Sadler's blog to be interesting and current. She uses thorough medical research and presents them in a manner in which we can all understand. By using real life patient experiences and family situations, she brings the topics to us in a personal way. Items both common and vaguely familiar often become relative to our everyday lives. Her blog leaves me feeling informed and, more importantly, entertained."

– Mike Richardson, Former NFL running back, SMU Hall of Fame

OPEN THIS BOOK AND SAY "AHHH"

A family practice doctor combines sound medical advice with a touch of humor

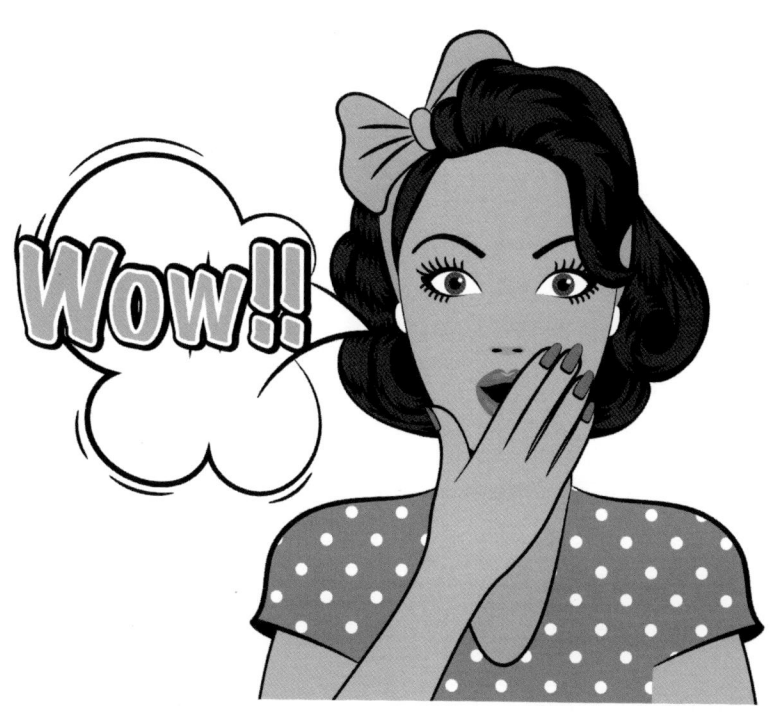

Jane Sadler, M.D.

Copyright © 2016 Dr. Jane Sadler

All Rights Reserved. No part of this publication may be reproduced, stored in a retrieval system, or transmitted, in any form or in any means—by electronic, mechanical, photocopying, recording or otherwise—without prior written permission.

ISBN#978-0-692-60114-3

Dr. Sadler's opinions and writings do not reflect those of Baylor Scott & White Health.

Author Photos by Brynn Rogers Photography

Printed in Canada

DEDICATION

A few years ago, I was invited to speak to graduating family-practice resident physicians. The young doctors wanted to hear about my family, my upbringing and my decision to become a doctor. They were also curious to know how I balanced family time with community service and a thriving medical practice. With honor and humility I stepped up to the podium, dedicating my speech to my parents and my love for the Lord.

I grew up in a dual-physician household. My parents were immigrants. My father, who was born in Egypt, had lost his mother when he was 14 and was raised by his brothers. He attended medical school and did his residency in Egypt while living in a hotel. Despite graduating at the top of his class, he could not get the hospital faculty position he desired, as his Christian Coptic religion was not looked upon favorably. He left for England, where the British medical community embraced him and he worked as a physician fellow, immersing himself in medical research.

While in England, Dad met my mother, an anesthesiology resident. She was the only girl in a family of five children and the only one to attend college. She had grown up during World War II, was "painfully shy" and had developed an awkward stutter, perhaps the result of having to attend 11 different schools prior to graduating from high school. (Multiple moves were necessary to avoid mandatory relocation during the Nazi bombings.)

Her family finally settled in Skegness, where they opened the Links Hotel, equipped with a full-service pub and a private closet in a telephone booth that hid contraband rationed beef. My mom, underage by today's standards, worked in the pub and was expected by her older brothers to serve drunken patrons. She named me after her favorite horse, Jane, which her father had received as a payment on a gambling debt.

Mumsie, my grandmother and the family matriarch, made certain Mom did not learn to cook because she wanted my mother to focus on school and a promising career outside the home. (Later, Mom's unfortunate lack of valuable kitchen skills, in combination with her busy work schedule, resulted in our family eating lots of TV dinners and Chef Boyardee.) While dating Dad, my mother was able to help him type his latest endocrinology research findings and thesis for his Ph.D. Mom found it a tedious two-finger job, but her exceptional writing skills enabled my father's broken English to find a home on paper.

After my father had completed his M.D.-Ph.D., he, my pregnant mother and my two older sisters traveled across the pond to the U.S., where Dad was invited to become a member of the physician faculty at Case Western Reserve University in Cleveland, Ohio.

It wasn't long before American generosity overwhelmed my parents. Very poor immigrants when they arrived in the States, my mother, pregnant with her third child (me), had secured a tiny, third-floor apartment downtown. Without a paycheck until the end of the month, Mom had less than $10 for the remaining weeks. She prayed to God for help.

God listened. Inside the one-bedroom apartment was an oversized American refrigerator. Opening its door, she was caught off guard by the overwhelming amount of food contained within its vast space. The landlady, seeing the scarcity of our family's belongings, had taken pity on us. My travel-weary, homesick mother fell to her knees in thanksgiving.

I was born a few months later. Both the obstetrician and the pediatrician made it clear that I would be significantly mentally and probably physically delayed. My mother refused to listen and prayed intently. She continued to pray daily for me and worked diligently to advance my physical and intellectual development. I did not speak for three years and did not walk until I was almost 3. The pediatrician remained guarded about my condition; my mother prayed with even more purpose. One night, at a friend's dinner party, I rose to my feet and began running. You see, my mother's daily prayers and her conviction and trust in the Lord set me free from my constraints and healed me.

    I thank her and I thank my God, and I dedicate this book to them.

With love to my low-carb, high-protein husband, John; my gluten-free daughter, Samantha; and my always hungry, carb-loving pizza man, son John Michael.

To my father: I really never minded when you called me your Baby Jane.

Sending appreciation to my mother, Jean. You encouraged me in everything.

TABLE OF CONTENTS

FRUCTOSE VS. GLUCOSE: A QUICK GUIDE FOR YOUR NEW YEAR'S RESOLUTION (OR ANYTIME) 15
NEW INFORMATION TO PROTECT YOUR BRAIN HEALTH 17
TRUST YOUR DOCTOR AND LEAVE THE RHINOCEROS ALONE! 19
COME IN HEALTHY, LEAVE WITH THE FLU 21
JUICING MAY PUT YOU AT RISK FOR DIABETES 23
CHRONIC COUGH CAUSING CONCERN? 25
HOW CAN YOU STAY SLIM AFTER EATING 32 DONUTS? 27
I AM SO EXCITED YOU LOST WEIGHT, BUT... 29
WHEN THE DOCTOR BECOMES THE PATIENT 31
WHO SAYS MEDICAL BILLING CAN'T BE FUNNY? 33
TOO CAUTIOUS WITH FOOD ALLERGIES? YOU MAY BE DOING MORE HARM THAN GOOD 35
WHY MOST DOCTORS CHOOSE TO DIE DIFFERENTLY FROM THEIR PATIENTS 38
I LOVE CHEETOS! AM I ADDICTED? 40
IS CLEANLINESS A CAUSE FOR ILLNESS? 42
YOU SNOOZE, YOU MAY LOSE...WEIGHT 44
INFANTILE COLIC MAY BE LINKED TO CHILDHOOD MIGRAINE 46
CONSTITUTIONAL LESSONS FROM MY DOG APPLIED TO YOUR DAILY CONSTITUTION 48

- WALK, DON'T RUN. IT'S THE DISTANCE THAT COUNTS 50
- PEPPERS ARE A NEW HOT TOPIC IN THE PREVENTION OF PARKINSON'S DISEASE 52
- EXERCISE TO GAIN 'GOOD' FAT AND RAISE YOUR METABOLISM 54
- FEEL SUPER ABOUT YOUR STATIN SAFETY 55
- IS LACK OF ESTROGEN KILLING YOU? 57
- 5 THINGS DOCTORS MAY NOT TELL YOU 59
- LABOR INDUCTION MAY BE LINKED TO AUTISM 62
- IT'S OK TO GO NUTS OVER COCONUT WATER 64
- POSTPARTUM PSYCHOSIS IS NOT THE BABY BLUES 65
- CELEBRATE STATINS! REDUCE DEMENTIA RISKS UP TO 3-FOLD 68
- LIVER FAILURE FROM A DIET SUPPLEMENT; BE CAREFUL 70
- KNOW THE 8 SYMPTOMS OF DEPRESSION 72
- YOU DON'T HAVE TO LOOK OR SOUND LIKE DARTH VADER TO HAVE SLEEP APNEA 74
- DON'T STUFF YOURSELF AT THANKSGIVING DINNER 76
- ARE YOUR REUSABLE GROCERY BAGS MAKING YOU SICK? 78
- YOUR KITCHEN SPONGE IS A GERM MAGNET 79
- SANTA, DON'T FALL ASLEEP IN YOUR SLEIGH 81
- DO YOU REALLY 'KNEE'D' SURGERY? 85
- 5 REASONS TO NOT BLOW OFF YOUR FLU SHOT 88
- I VACUUMED MY DOG TODAY 90
- REDUCING FEVER MAY PROLONG OR WORSEN FLU 91

WHAT SHOULD YOU TAKE FOR THAT PESKY COLD?	93
8 REASONS WHY ALL CALORIES ARE NOT THE SAME	96
I LOVE EAU DE MOO! WHY DON'T YOU?	98
IS YOUR TEEN ADDICTED TO HIS OR HER PHONE?	100
EXERCISE IS A YEAR-ROUND SPORT	103
$1,000 A MONTH ON SUPPLEMENTS	105
IS YOUR DIET SODA KILLING YOU?	107
ARE ANTI-AGING HORMONES AGING YOU?	109
CAN THAT CUP OF JOE HELP YOU LOSE YOUR MUFFIN TOP?	111
BEWARE OF BAMBOO BONFIRES AND RABID FERRET-BADGERS!	113
WILL IT TAKE YOUNGER BLOOD TO MAKE YOUR BRAIN FEEL YOUTHFUL?	115
7 WAYS NOT TO TREAT A SNAKE BITE	117
SHOULD YOU REALLY 'DRINK' TO GOOD SKIN HEALTH?	119
DO YOU 'KNEE-D' MORE MILK?	121
I CUT MY FINGER AND FOUND 6 STEPS FOR MORE RAPID WOUND CARE	123
GODZILLA SPREADING SALMONELLA IN NEW YORK CITY	125
WHY YOU SHOULD BE 'THAT GIRL' (OR GUY)!	127
YOUR DOCTOR MAY SEE A PROBLEM WITH YOUR CHILD'S WEIGHT	129
WHAT DOES ELEVATED BLOOD SUGAR HAVE TO DO WITH CANCER?	131
ARTIFICIAL SWEETENERS: TRUST YOUR GUT	133
IS THERE A VIRUS INSIDE US? MOST LIKELY, YES!	135

5 SURPRISING HEALTH BENEFITS OF COFFEE 137

10 TIPS FOR TACKLING ACUTE BACK PAIN 139

YOU MAY NOT BE ALLERGIC TO PENICILLIN 142

TIME FOR YOUR PHYSICAL! BUT WHAT IF YOUR DOCTOR FINDS SOMETHING WRONG? 145

POOR TEXTING POSTURE IS A PAIN IN THE NECK 147

HOLIDAY FEASTS MAY LEAD TO 'HOLIDAY HEART' 149

MULTITASKING IS BAD FOR THE BRAIN (AND MY DAUGHTER'S IPHONE) 151

WANT THE NEW YEAR TO BEGIN HEALTHIER? THINK YOGURT! 153

EGG-CITING NEWS FOR PEOPLE WHO LOVE EGGS 155

BREAKING HEALTHY 157

HOW COLD? EQUESTRIAN PANNICULITIS COLD! 160

IS THERE A DOCTOR ON THE PLANE? (OR, MEDICAL CONDITIONS THAT DON'T FLY WELL) 162

A CLUTTERED ROOM AND A CLUTTERED MIND 164

WHAT DO BROKEN MIRRORS AND HOT FLASHES HAVE IN COMMON? 7 HOT FLASH FACTS 165

BATS BITE IN THE SPRING (NOT JUST HALLOWEEN) 167

8 SIGNS THAT YOUR HEALTHY EATING IS MAKING YOU SICK 169

SOME FATS ARE NOT ALL THAT BAD AND SOME ARE THE BEE'S KNEES! 171

10 LIFE-SAVING FACTS YOU NEED TO KNOW ABOUT LIGHTNING 173

ARE YOU ITCHING TO GET OUT IN THE SUN, OR DOES THE SUN MAKE YOU ITCH? 175

DO YOU ATTRACT OR REPEL MOSQUITOES? 7 HELPFUL MOSQUITO FACTS 177

7 SOUR TRUTHS ABOUT SWEETENED BEVERAGES 180

YOU MAY BE 1 OF THE 13 MILLION TO BENEFIT FROM THIS NEWS	182
SPICE IT UP AND ADD YEARS TO YOUR LIFE	184
PARENTING DOES NOT HAVE TO BE A TRAUMATIC EXPERIENCE	186
7 REFRIGERATOR-WORTHY HEALTHY HABITS TO MAINTAIN YOUR STUDENT'S HEALTH	188
HAND SANITIZING: SKIP THE SCRUB AND GO FOR THE SQUIRT?	190
4 NONFICTION FACTS FOR 4 FLU FOLKTALES	192
SHRINK ABOUT IT: PRESCRIPTION ESTROGEN WITH DIABETES	194
SKIP THE SUPPLEMENT: FISH ARE FRIENDS AND FOOD	196
5 MYTHS AND 5 RECOVERY TOOLS FOR CELEBRATING THE NEW YEAR	198
ARE STETHOSCOPES GOING THE WAY OF THE TYPEWRITER, OR JUST AGING GRACEFULLY?	201
DOES A FULL MOON AFFECT YOUR MOOD? TRUTH BE TOLD	203
GOT PERIMENOPAUSE? STIMULATE YOUR SKIN TO KEEP IT SMOOTHER	205
DON'T BURY YOUR HEAD IN THE SAND; ENJOY THE BEACH	207
CALORIES DON'T COUNT WHEN I STEAL THEM OFF YOUR PLATE	210
MY COLD HAS GONE VIRAL!	212
WHAT TO DO WHEN YOU HAVE THE STOMACH FLU	214
ABOUT THE AUTHOR	217

These blogs were written between 2013 and 2016 and are presented in the order they were written.

FRUCTOSE VS. GLUCOSE: A QUICK GUIDE FOR YOUR NEW YEAR'S RESOLUTION (OR ANYTIME)

I am certain that most people have "weight loss" at the top of their list of New Year's resolutions. But why should I take time to explain why it matters which sweetener you choose? For many reasons.

Significant differences exist in how the sugars fructose and glucose are metabolized by the body. Research from the Journal of the American Medical Association (January 2013) seems to indicate that fructose reduces brain activity and may adversely affect the brain's appetite and reward pathways. Fructose and other sugars possibly increase "food-seeking behavior" and food intake.

A Journal of Clinical Investigation study (2009) also demonstrated important differences in how fructose and glucose are metabolized. Over 10 weeks men and women drank either glucose- or fructose-sweetened beverages, totaling 25 percent of their daily calorie intake. Both groups gained weight, but imaging studies revealed that the fructose group tended to gain more belly fat while the glucose group added fat under the skin (subcutaneous fat).

Belly fat has been linked to heart disease and liver disease. LDL "bad cholesterol" and triglycerides (fats) were also elevated in the fructose group, adding to concerns that diets high in fructose may promote diabetes over time. On the other hand, excess subcutaneous fat (fat underneath the skin) was not associated with a higher risk for developing diabetes (Journal of the American Medical Association, September 2012).

But how is fructose different from glucose? Fructose is found (blended) with sucrose in table sugar, corn syrup, high fructose corn syrup, crystalline fructose, concentrated fruit juices, and natural sweeteners such as honey and agave. Glucose is another kind of simple sugar that is found in starches and in about 50 percent of table sugar (the other 50 percent is fructose). Glucose plus fructose are commonly referred to as sucrose (a disaccharide sugar, meaning it is made up of two monosaccharide sugar units).

So, fructose is very difficult to avoid if you prefer sweetened foods and beverages. Be wary of "healthy" fruit beverages you buy at the grocery store or coffee bar. Sources of fructose include sweetened beverages and soft drinks. When you read nutrition labels, high fructose corn syrup is commonly one of the first items listed and therefore a significant addition to whatever it is you are about to eat. Avoid it as much as possible and choose natural foods that are not processed, such as whole fruits (with non-processed or concentrated levels of fructose) and vegetables.

Be more sophisticated in your New Year's resolutions. When looking through the health food aisle, make wise choices. Avoid sugary drinks. Even "natural" juices can be significant poor-health choices. If you are thirsty, drink water (unsweetened). One life. One body. Take care of it! ☛

NEW INFORMATION TO PROTECT YOUR BRAIN HEALTH

I heard on the ABC morning show today that beta blockers (a blood pressure medication) may reduce the risk of Alzheimer's disease. That is great and interesting news released from the American Academy of Neurology's annual meeting, and super food for my blog today. But the main meal comes from a 2007 article in the Journal of Neurology, Neurosurgery & Psychiatry. According to this study, another class of commonly used blood pressure medications and cholesterol lowering medications can significantly decrease the progression of Alzheimer's disease.

Blood pressure medications that work on the renin-angiotensin system (kidney) and statin drugs (such as Lipitor) could certainly lower the risk of deterioration of dementia. I LOVE to blog on the benefits of statin drugs for high cholesterol and always get a smile on my face when more information about the benefits of statin drugs are released.

Just as important as the benefits of beta blockers and statins are the potential issues related to long-term use of anti-anxiety medications (anxiolytics). Now pay attention, because here comes dessert: Drugs that control acute anxiety and psychosis can lead to acceleration of Alzheimer's.* Anxiolytics such as Xanax and Valium (benzodiazepine class) may contribute significantly to the decline in brain activity associated with dementia. When added to anti-psychotics (e.g., Haldol and Risperdal), anxiolytics can lead to even more significant deterioration of memory. Interestingly, anti-depressants like Prozac had no adverse effects on the progression of Alzheimer's disease.

High quality of life is very important as we become an aging population, so be sure you are paying attention to this information, and use it to your advantage! If your blood pressure is high, get it treated and discuss with your doctor medications that have "healthy-brain options." Don't be afraid of medications that could lower your blood pressure and potentially improve brain health. If you have anxiety or suffer from psychosis (such as schizophrenia), you and your doctor should carefully weigh the risks and benefits of all your medications. There are many options for safe, long-term treatment. ☛

*"The effects of commonly prescribed drugs in patients with Alzheimer's disease on the rate of deterioration," Journal of Neurology, Neurosurgery & Psychiatry, March 2007

WHAT DO WE REALLY "SEE" IN SEAFOOD?

I love to write about the benefits of seafood. But this information concerned me. Consumer Reports conducted DNA testing of sushi from sushi bars, restaurants and grocery stores. The evaluation, of 119 fish samples, found that 55% were mislabeled. Red snapper was misidentified 100% of the time. In 21 sushi restaurants in Los Angeles, mislabeling occurred in 87% of fish samples.

TRUST YOUR DOCTOR AND LEAVE THE RHINOCEROS ALONE!

Really? Do you really believe that using rhinoceros horn is going to improve your sex life, cure your cancer or improve your health in any other way? Really?

I had to unclench my jaw after reading about the $500,000 worth of rhino horns seized from a Bangkok airport. The needless slaughter of rare and precious animals for purposes of "natural" medical remedies puts rocks in my gut. I have no patience for this level of thinking.

Rhinoceros horn contains keratin, which is found in hair, fingernails and animal hooves. A single rhinoceros horn can be valued at up to $25,000. The price for this precious commodity is reaching above $1,660 per gram, more than the price of gold! Why does material the equivalent of tough toenails reach such ridiculous values?

Some cultures believe the rhinoceros horn can cure anything from cancer to the common cold. The ancient Persians (of the 5th century B.C.) thought that bowls carved from the horn could be used to detect poisoned liquids. The belief persisted into the 18th and 19th centuries among the royal courts of Europe, according to PBS show *Nature*. If a liquid placed in the rhinoceros horn vessel produced a "bubbling" reaction, it was thought to reveal poisonous material.

I scoured for any proof of the horn's healing properties. The only evidence I found was research done in 1990 at a Chinese university in Hong Kong that found that large amounts of rhino horn could slightly lower fever in rats. The large amount of horn given in the Chinese experiments was, however, far greater than the amount generally used in typical Chinese medicine. In other words, if you chose rhino horn to treat a low-grade fever, you would need to take out a bank loan.

Please don't sacrifice the rhinoceros—use acetaminophen or ibuprofen instead, and trust your doctor to help you take care of your other medical problems. Rhinoceros horns do not improve sex drive or cure asthma, arthritis or cancer. Choose modern, sophisticated medicine and avoid fairy tales that proclaim miracle cures from this endangered animal. There are only about 25,000 rhinos left in the wild. For information on how you can save rhinos from extinction, go to savetherhino.org. ☛

COME IN HEALTHY, LEAVE WITH THE FLU

Some people may consider it job security (we doctors do not), but when you come for a well check (a physical) you may be getting more than what you bargained for: the flu. This is especially true during this unusually active flu season.

Two patients I saw last week developed flu-like symptoms within 24-48 hours of their office visits. Symptoms included high fever, cough, muscle aches and runny nose. We can only hope Tamiflu (to treat flu) is still available at the local pharmacy.

My advice for patients who have scheduled well checks/physicals (blood pressure check, cholesterol testing, etc.) in the next several weeks is to consider rescheduling your appointment if you have no urgent concerns. For example, if your blood pressure has done well and you do not suffer uncontrolled diabetes or other problems, think about contacting your physician to determine if delaying your physical is a reasonable option.

If you bring in a sick child, don't bring your healthy children, too. Find someone (if you can) to care for your healthy children so that they can avoid the contagion within the medical office.

At my clinic, we have remained unusually busy this flu season, although the number of flu cases seem to be leveling off. In the U.S., flu has killed 20 children so far this season, according to the CDC (Centers for Disease Control and Prevention), and vaccine shortages have been announced.

In the office Monday, I saw an 18-month-old boy who could not receive his flu shot because my office didn't have enough vaccine. A friend texted me Friday requesting nasal flu vaccines for her family, and I had none to give her. So sorry. I am down to nothing and have heard no news about the near-future availability of the flu vaccine.

But you may still be able to get your flu shot. Take a look at flu.gov for information about the availability of flu vaccine in your community.

If you do not suffer from a chronic disease, reschedule your well visit if your doctor agrees. But get to the office quickly if you develop fever, runny nose, cough or muscle aches, and get treated and get well. ☛

JUICING MAY PUT YOU AT RISK FOR DIABETES

I get my blog ideas from daily experiences and put my blogs together during my daily dog walks. There is something so refreshing about being outside after a day cooped up at the office.

Tonight was very cold and my walk was short, therefore so is my blog. But please read this blog if you are engaged in any non-medically supervised diet. The extent healthy young people will go to in order to rapidly lose unwanted pounds can negatively impact their health.

Elevated blood sugars in an otherwise healthy adult patient on a juicing diet raised my level of concern for this popular diet craze. The high-fructose corn syrup in concentrated blended juices and a family history of diabetes was what triggered us to check "Sam's" blood sugars. This 23-year-old had a glucose (blood sugar) level that was significantly elevated approximately two hours after eating. Untreated, persistently elevated blood sugars define diabetes, which is a disease that can damage the blood vessels, kidneys, eyes and heart.

"Juicing," or drinking liquids with concentrated fresh fruits, may cause significant spikes in blood sugars after eating. While for many healthy people that may not be terrible, for others it could result in repeated stress on the pancreas to secrete bolus (concentrated and large) amounts of insulin. Insulin helps to move glucose into the body for use as energy. As the body gets used to these sugar boluses, it may require more and more insulin in order to move glucose into the muscles and organs. In other words, much like a drug addict requiring increasing amounts of narcotics to maintain his "high," more and more insulin is needed over time to meet the growing needs of the sugar load (American Diabetes Association's Diabetes Care journal, January 2008 and January 2013).

If you're a "juicer," you may not know whether this information applies to you. Do yourself a favor and check your two-hour post-prandial blood sugar after juicing. What this involves is a finger stick for blood sugar two hours after your juicing experience (or whatever you call it). Your blood sugar should be less than 140 milligrams/deciliter (mg/dL) if you are age 50 or younger; less than 150 for ages 50-60; and less than 160mg/dL for ages 60 or older.

You would be surprised how many patients I see with prediabetes. Patients whose sugars are borderline high and who continue to ingest concentrated fruit drinks may develop diabetes unless they adopt a healthier lifestyle. Studies in Diabetes Care have reaffirmed my concerns. Choosing to eat whole fruits and vegetables is a slower and more appetite-fulfilling process. Yes, "you could've had a V-8," but wouldn't it be more satisfying to finish off an entire carrot, a few leafy vegetables and a pear?

CHRONIC COUGH CAUSING CONCERN?

That post-flu cough is not going away anytime soon. You thought you "nailed it" by beginning Tamiflu early in the course of the infection. Of course, you felt better faster than if you had delayed seeking treatment for the flu. But despite the fact that you are feeling so much better, the cough has been lingering for almost two weeks. It must be time for antibiotics, right?

No. Most coughs associated with respiratory illnesses (including the flu) may take an average of 18 days to resolve, according to a January 2013 study in the Annals of Family Medicine journal. If you are feeling well other than the cough, you should just try to wait it out and see if the cough goes away on its own. However, recognize these alarm symptoms that should trigger a visit to your doctor:

- Fever (greater than 100.4 F)
- Vomiting
- Shortness of breath
- Bloody productive cough
- Wheezing
- Chest pain

Especially when it comes to children, physicians are intensely trying to cut back on antibiotic use in situations of cough. We have learned from earlier studies, including one from the Clinical & Experimental Allergy journal (1999) linking antibiotic use in the first year of life to an increased likelihood of childhood asthma. Today, I saw an otherwise healthy infant who (elsewhere) had been prescribed antibiotics for a few days of cough. Mom came in for a second opinion. A thorough evaluation including blood count and chest x-ray made it quite clear this illness was viral in nature. Viral infections do NOT respond to antibiotics, and antibiotics would not change the course of this particular illness. With close follow-up, we should be able to avoid antibiotic use in this baby. Because of her young age, I'll see her again tomorrow to be sure she is doing well.

Additionally, not all coughs are from the respiratory tract (sinuses and lungs). Coughs may be caused by side effects of certain blood pressure medications, allergies or even acid reflux. It is important that if your cough is associated with alarm symptoms (listed above), you seek evaluation and treatment by your physician.

HOW CAN YOU STAY SLIM AFTER EATING 32 DONUTS?

32 donuts! That's how many Uncle Si ate in a family donut-eating contest on a recent episode of Duck Dynasty. 32 donuts! He sat down at the counter and ate 32 donuts (sorry, I am still going through stages of disbelief).

This is not the first time Uncle Si has been in the spotlight. In a prior episode, the family poked fun at him for his frequent trips to the restroom. While house hunting, he repeatedly had to leave his interview to find bladder relief in a nearby restroom. Hmm...the hamster in my brain is turning the cycling wheels a bit faster now...what is really going on here? Let me try to put this information together.

Based on my medical training and professional viewing experience of Duck Dynasty, I am highly concerned that Uncle Si has diabetes. Polyuria (frequent urination), polyphagia (increased appetite) and low weight are all suggestive of high blood sugars. He is suspiciously slim for someone who can eat 32 (32!) donuts in one sitting.

But Uncle Si is not alone in presenting symptoms consistent with diabetes. About two or three times a year a patient comes to my office for a routine evaluation and has unexplained weight loss. Before I congratulate him on losing excess pounds, I take a good look at his general health. Muscle wasting (atrophy) and poor skin tone may be signs of unhealthy weight loss due to prolonged elevated blood sugars. When the body is unable to use available blood sugar, glucose (sugar) is excreted through the kidneys along with vital nutrients and protein, resulting in loss of energy to the organs of the body. The result is severe physical compromise of the organs including muscles, kidneys, heart, etc. Over time, the person will take on an unhealthy appearance. Uncle Si does not have a healthy appearance (and I am not talking about his scraggly beard).

Of course, other problems could cause unexplained weight loss, such as cancer, drug use and metabolic hyper-metabolism (high thyroid, for example). I would suggest that anyone who eats 32 donuts at one sitting, has frequent urination and low body weight seek professional evaluation with his or her physician. Uncle Si, come on over! I would love to take a good look at your general health and give you an expert opinion.

I AM SO EXCITED YOU LOST WEIGHT, BUT...

I am so excited that you lost 50 pounds. Your blood pressure, cholesterol, blood sugar and pulse are also down. I am pleased you did not require weight loss surgery in order to take off unhealthy pounds. I am very glad you found a weight loss program that works for you, but please do not ask me to review piles of information, sell or promote it over any other solutions available for my patients. Yesterday it was "the gluten-free diet" and the Isagenix diet, and today it is the "addicted-brain diet." There are many methods to lose weight; I am just so glad you found one that works for you.

When we spoke last year, we discussed the necessity of weight loss in order to preserve a healthier retirement. Losing weight could decrease the possibility of spending your important retirement dollars on clinic, lab and hospital visits.

We discussed that any method that involves lower daily calories that you could adhere to relatively easily would be a good fit. You found a method, and I am ecstatic. It makes my job as your physician much easier (I know, very selfish of me) because your overall health care is easier to manage when you control your own hypertension, high cholesterol and blood sugar.

Studies show time and again that less calorie intake equals less weight. People do not have to spend a lot of money to understand that concept. Nonetheless, many weight loss programs include a little more "hand-holding," which definitely adds to successful results. I cannot, however, recommend your program over any other, but if the program works best for YOU and has proven, long-lasting results, then it is YOUR best fit.

Purchasing multivitamins, supplements, shakes and books does not guarantee weight loss. It is your personal "buy-in" to a program that fits your lifestyle and can work best for you. So, keep up the good work. Encourage family, friends and neighbors to live healthier lives and lose unnecessary pounds. But please understand, I cannot promote the many, many diet programs that come to my attention.

WHEN THE DOCTOR BECOMES THE PATIENT

"Your blood sugar is too high" was my doctor's report. The words hit me like a ton of bricks, and my thoughts quickly tumbled out of control. I may have diabetes. I need to begin checking blood sugars. What medication will work best for me? How could this happen? I had some unintentional weight loss recently, but I chalked that up to a vigorous work schedule.

Then a flashback. Although I am slim and in good physical condition, I had eaten five pounds (yes, five pounds) of Smarties candies during my last pregnancy and at the time was chastised by my obstetrician when he noticed sugar in my urine (sometimes the first sign of diabetes). Adding to my concern is my family history of diabetes. My father had diabetes and died of its complications due to his delay in seeking treatment.

According to the ADA (American Diabetes Association), approximately 25.8 million Americans have diabetes, and about 7 million of them do not know it. Diabetes is the number one cause of blindness and kidney failure in the United States, and diabetes is preventable in up to 95 percent of cases, according to a recent report from the Archives of Internal Medicine. If you do have prediabetes (borderline diabetes), there is a 58 percent chance you can avoid diabetes with excellent lifestyle choices. The lifestyle choice with the biggest impact: weight loss.

To finish my story, I did go back for additional testing. Under my doctor's strict guidance, I had my hemoglobin A1c test performed. This test reveals the three-month average of blood sugars and is a highly sensitive test for diabetes. My number was low…real good.

Then, I remembered I had had a latte with extra cream just prior to my initial lab draw and was not truly "fasting" (without food intake). OK. I feel better. But, lessons learned and a wake-up call. Diabetes is a preventable disease. Take charge of your health. ☛

> Hope you didn't miss National Pie Day, which is Jan. 23. Several restaurants were offering free pie slices. Sorry, as your doctor, I cannot recommend regular doses of pie, but occasionally a little bit here and there can temporarily raise "feel-good" chemicals in the brain, and on National Pie Day it is just what this doctor prescribes!

WHO SAYS MEDICAL BILLING CAN'T BE FUNNY?

I don't find medical billing to be humorous at all. I never smile or laugh when I get my receipt for medical charges in the mail. As a physician leader, I sit on a medical-coding compliance committee and we rarely have anything "juicy" to discuss. In fact (sorry to all my committee members), sometimes it can be downright boring. What is so exciting about billing for respiratory infections, hypertension or diabetes? Nothing!

But at our last meeting I almost fell out of my chair laughing. One of our members brought in a list of new billing codes for potential use in the medical encounter. These funny codes remind me that family practice is like a "box of chocolates"—you never know WHAT you are going to get when you walk into the exam room.

Here are some diagnosis codes with billing numbers your physician could use just in case you experience strange (or hilarious) situations:

- Walked into a lamppost, initial encounter (W22.02XA)
- Injured knitting and crocheting (E012.0)
- Burn injury due to water skis on fire, initial encounter (V91.07XA)
- Struck by turtle, initial encounter (W59.22)

   I can't make these up...

- Struck by duck, initial encounter (W61.62XA)
- Contact with duck (W61.1)

- Activity, ironing (Y93.E4)
- Squash court as place of occurrence of the external cause (Y92.311) (Huh?)
- Spacecraft collision injuring participant (V95.43)
- Crushed by alligator, initial encounter (W5803XA)
- Accidental mechanical suffocation by falling earth or other substance (E913.3)
- Bizarre personal appearance (R46.1)
- Discord with boss and workmates (Z56.4)
- Type A personality (Z732)
- Lack of relaxation and leisure (Z73.2)
- Chicken coop as the place of occurrence of the external cause (Y92.72)

So, be certain (your government at work) that your doctor has access to billing codes for anything that might occur. Just don't try the above maneuvers without physician supervision and medical care. Also, avoid chicken coops! ☛

TOO CAUTIOUS WITH FOOD ALLERGIES? YOU MAY BE DOING MORE HARM THAN GOOD

Throughout my professional career as a physician, I have been taught to spare children exposure to allergenic foods such as peanuts, shrimp and eggs until they are older. In fact, long-standing recommendations from the American Academy of Pediatrics have had physicians discourage parents from introducing milk until age 1, eggs until age 2 and peanuts until a child is 3.

Overprotecting children may be harmful, however, when it comes to food allergies. Consider results from a recent study that found that British Jewish children were 10 times more likely than Israeli Jewish children to have a peanut allergy. The Israeli kids are exposed early in life to a diet rich in nuts; some are given peanut-laden foods at just a few months of age. British children are generally not exposed to nuts until 1 year of age.

According to the National Institute of Allergy and Infectious Diseases, the incidence of food allergies in children increased by 18 percent between 1997 and 2007. About 5 percent of children in the United States under age 5 have food allergies. Based on several studies, the American Academy of Allergy, Asthma & Immunology (AAAAI), in a Journal of Allergy and Clinical Immunology report, has made an "about-face" in recommendations of when to introduce highly allergic foods to babies. According to the AAAAI, foods that should be introduced early in infancy include wheat, soy, milk, tree nuts and shellfish (yes, shellfish!).

One theory (which explains why early "highly allergenic" food introduction is important) is that it becomes necessary for a baby's immune system to be exposed during a "critical window" around 4-6 months of age when the child first starts to eat solids, according to Dr. Katie Allen, professor at Royal Children's Hospital in Australia. In addition, we may be overly clean in preventing exposure to allergens and germs in our children. Potentially, this could compromise the development of their immune system. The Wall Street Journal (March 4, 2014) has written a wonderful article summarizing these studies.

In addition, we need to look at our basic child nutrition. There are studies that link food allergies and vitamin D, including one from the Journal of Allergy and Clinical Immunology, which discovered that low vitamin D levels in 5,000 babies was associated with up to a three times higher likelihood of food allergies. Very impressive, as a 2009 article in the journal Pediatrics estimated that approximately 20 percent of children in the United States might be vitamin D deficient.

So what do we do with this information? Should we be concerned about introducing these allergenic foods to our children? What if they have a severe reaction? Up to 39 percent of children with food allergies do have a severe reaction, according to a 2011 report in the journal Pediatrics. However, the AAAAI now recommends introducing the allergic foods to a baby just after typical first foods are tolerated. Begin with rice cereal, fruits and vegetables, then gradually introduce nuts, eggs, etc., in increasing amounts.

The AAAAI does recommend caution and possible referral to an allergy physician in cases where an infant has severe eczema (skin allergies) or a sibling with a peanut allergy (risk of allergy to nuts is approximately 7 percent in these kids). As always, I recommend you consult with your personal physician prior to introducing allergenic foods to your babies.

As a parent and physician, I understand the meaning of being overprotective, but it is hard to let go of previous strict diet standards for our babies. Perhaps the paradox is that being too cautious may do more harm in the case of food sensitivities, and we should all allow more variety and less restraint in dietary choices.

Personally, I love seafood, nuts and soybeans and I love to boast the health benefits of the Mediterranean diet. Introducing these colorful foods into your regular meals will positively impact the heart health of future generations. ☛

> Feb. 5 is the day to greet your favorite weather forecaster with pancakes dipped in chocolate fondue sauce. It is National Pancake Day, National Weatherman's Day and National Chocolate Fondue Day. Celebrate this day!

WHY MOST DOCTORS CHOOSE TO DIE DIFFERENTLY FROM THEIR PATIENTS

My blog today is based on reading a commentary by Michael Pistoria, in Family Practice News. He comments on a Feb. 25, 2012, article from the *Wall Street Journal* in which author Dr. Ken Murray reviews physicians' personal decisions regarding their own end-of-life care. "Why should doctors die differently?" Dr. Pistoria asks.

According to the article, 800 physicians who graduated between 1948 and 1964 from Johns Hopkins were surveyed in the early 2000s. Advanced directives had been created by 64 percent of the physicians, compared with 20 percent of the general public.

An advanced directive lets your family know what level of medical care you would want if you were unable to make the decision on your own. For example, if you were in a coma and on continual need for life-support, would you want ongoing medical care if there was no hope of recovery?

Reference to a patient's advanced directive is an important standard we physicians use in order to ensure our patient is medically managed according to his or her wishes. Knowing a patient's personal decision in advance of a tragedy helps the family abide by their loved one's wishes. At times, it can be a patient's greatest legacy: maintaining peace within the family regarding decisions about ongoing medical care. The decision to withhold life support is an extraordinary one that should be discussed as far in advance as possible of any life-ending illness.

The survey written about in the WSJ found that almost 90 percent of the 800 physicians, compared to 25 percent of the general population, did not want CPR if they were in a chronic coma. This huge discrepancy may be explained by doctors' professional experiences in end-of-life decisions. So many times families innocently insist on ongoing, futile treatments that do not benefit the suffering of their loved ones. In patients with catastrophic strokes or injuries, it would be nice to know each patient's individual treatment decisions ahead of time. Many times, health care workers are left to assist CPR in situations that they may consider prolonging pain and suffering.

CPR (cardiopulmonary resuscitation) is an important skill to learn and put to work, but a 2010 study that evaluated the impact of 95,000 cases of CPR in Japan revealed that only 8 percent of patients survived for more than one month and only 3 percent of those went on to lead "normal" lives (I am not certain what "normal" means in these situations, as patients may have suffered significant brain injury as a result of the event that led to the need for CPR).

It is important for your physician to fully explain the medical options, risks and benefits of ongoing medical care and an advanced desire for CPR for you and your family members. Why should doctors choose to die differently? Perhaps you should discuss your end-of-life care openly with your physician. An advanced directive can be found on AMA-assn.org.

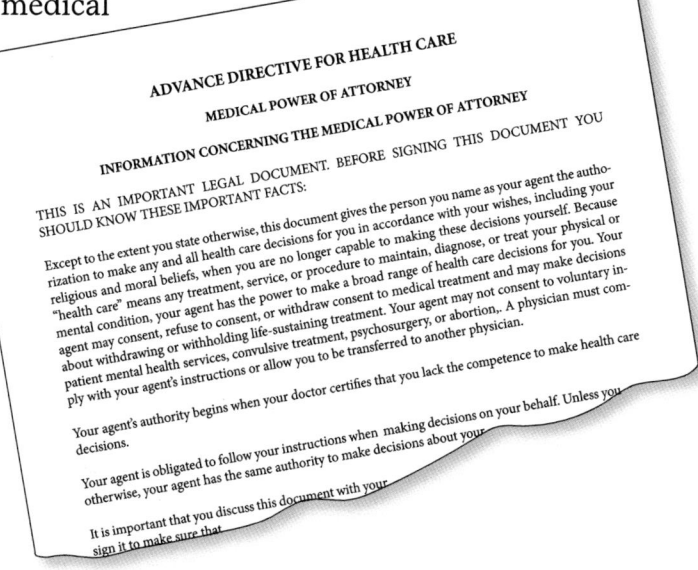

I LOVE CHEETOS! AM I ADDICTED?

I love Cheetos! Don't tell anyone (I think I already did), but I really do LOVE Cheetos! They are not good for me at all. Crammed with fats, salt and processed starches, they are the ULTIMATE bad food. I never eat Cheetos around anyone, and especially never at work, because Cheetos turn my fingers orange and that is highly embarrassing and unhygienic. Generally, I only eat Cheetos when I "steal" a few from my kids. I tell them it is their "kiddie tax" and that I am owed a certain percentage of the contents of their Cheetos bag.

Why do I love Cheetos? Because they are high in fats and salt. This indulgent snack is a favorite among teens and considered a highly palatable food, according to a 2010 article in Addiction about research at Yale. Studies show that rats consuming high levels of salt, sugars and fats have demonstrated increases in compulsive eating and consumption. Does this eating behavior mimic that of your teenagers?

Cheetos are addictive. In my favorite version of Cheetos—Flamin' Hot—one serving contains 10 grams of fat and 1/3 of our daily salt intake. The Rudd Center for Food Science and Policy compares urges for highly palatable food to urges for addictive drugs such as cocaine and heroin. Similar to the brain's activated response to addictive drugs, these foods stimulate the brain's reward and pleasure centers. Because foods like Cheetos are consumed earlier in life than addictive drugs, repeated exposure to highly palatable foods (like Cheetos) may lead to high levels of treatment-resistant food addiction. Be careful what you keep in your pantry. What kid doesn't like Cheetos?

So choose healthier foods for you and your family. I did find a bag of healthier baked Cheetos that only has 4.5 grams of fat and 8 percent of my daily salt intake. I think I could indulge in these Cheetos (with my dark chocolate) on rainy days. It is beginning to look a little overcast now... ☞

> A Detroit lady was suspected of having cancer when she went to the doctor with muscle and bone pain and was found to have abnormal mineral deposits in her bones. Because of these changes, her teeth were breaking and her bones were becoming brittle (putting her at high risk for fracture). Doctors discovered that her condition was caused by 17 years of drinking daily pitchers of tea made with 100 tea bags. Lucky for her, cutting back on her tea drinking will cure her problem. Remember, too much of a good thing can be bad.

IS CLEANLINESS A CAUSE FOR ILLNESS?

I admit, I am a closet clean-a-holic. Some would say I am a little obsessed with tidying up at my house. My mother hates it when I come to the ranch and start cleaning the floors. It's useless trying to keep that place sterile. People come in and out with dirt and cow dung stuck to the bottom of their boots. Chicken feathers and horse and dog hair coat the floors, and even the Dustbuster overheats trying to keep up with the mess.

Perhaps my futile efforts to clean are unnecessary. Today I have learned that my "OCD" cleaning issue (as my daughter calls it) may be having an adverse effect on my family's health. While cleaning is my effort to get rid of bacteria, fungi and insect waste, my family may need all these bugs in order to develop a better germ-fighting immune system.

A 2012 study of Amish children demonstrated lower levels of asthma, allergies and eczema (skin inflammation) in kids exposed to raw cow's milk. Apparently the exposure to natural bacteria found in raw milk (versus pasteurized milk) provided their bodies with stronger immunity to common allergens (grasses, trees, etc.). The "hygiene hypothesis" (David Strachen, 1989) is that kids exposed to a lot of germs early in life were less likely to become ill later in life. These findings are consistent with a study I previously cited from the American Academy of Pediatrics on dog exposure and decreased risk for respiratory infections during an infant's first year of life.

Does this mean I need to put down the mop, the sponge and the dish towel? What about the antibacterial gel that I obsessively thrust toward the kids to use before eating a meal?

In order to separate myself from clean, I will need some counseling and deconditioning for sure. For now, I will opt in for "cleanliness is next to godliness." But, if I were a parent of a newborn, I might think a little bit differently and relax my housekeeping efforts a bit. ☞

> **UNUSUAL MEDICAL BILLING CODES**
>
> **W55.21**
> **BITTEN BY A COW**
>
> *I have grown up with cows and have never known cows to bite.*

YOU SNOOZE, YOU MAY LOSE...WEIGHT

Are you having trouble losing weight? What if I told you that the more hours you sleep at night, the more likely you will lose pounds? Studies from University of Texas Southwestern here in Dallas have demonstrated that when the body is stressed due to inadequate sleep, it overcompensates with increased "energy" intake (i.e., calories).

But sleep is not just about the number of hours spent sleeping. It is also about the quality of sleep. Sleep apnea is a cause of poor-quality sleep. This is a condition in which lack of adequate oxygen intake during sleep can negatively impact the ability of the brain, heart and lungs to obtain healthy sleep. Obesity is a main cause of sleep apnea, and obesity can cause physical symptoms such as snoring and impose stress on these vital organs, increasing blood pressure and decreasing oxygenation to the brain at night.

Additionally, the physical strain of sleep apnea can elevate stress hormones such as cortisol, ghrelin and leptin, which affect appetite and hunger.

Studies out of Stanford University have shown that abnormalities of these levels as a result of sleep deprivation can have adverse effects on body fat and increase the risk for obesity.

Feeling tired and hungry is therefore NOT a good combination. Over time, the weight can pile on. It is a cyclic event that can lead to many problems, including increased blood pressure and heart disease.

So, can sleeping more help you lose weight? Scientists suggest that reducing stress hormones, which promote hunger, could be an adjunct to a reduced-calorie diet in successful weight loss. Reset your clock, get to bed earlier, and rest longer. Include at least eight hours of restful sleep in your diet plan because sleep deprivation could really be a "hunger-buster." ☛

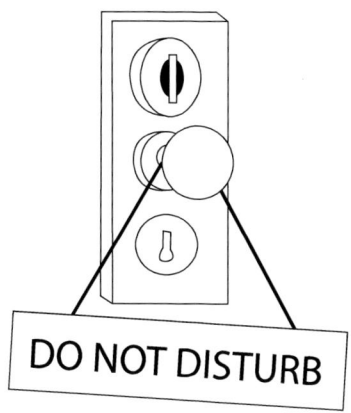

INFANTILE COLIC MAY BE LINKED TO CHILDHOOD MIGRAINE

My child had the worst infant colic. The inconsolable crying was so bad that everyone at church recognized her ID number when it flashed behind the pulpit. The congregation was keenly aware that the Sadler parents were being urgently notified to remove their child from the nursery. Her crying could have set off fire alarms it was so loud.

It did not matter that I took care of healthy, ill and needy infants in medical training and practice for many years prior to having children. I had spent countless nights awake in the newborn nursery and intensive care centers listening patiently to perpetually crying infants waiting to be healed and held. But I knew what was wrong with them...they were sick. I was a rock.

But no 48-hour call days could ever have prepared me for the nerve-racking task of managing my colicky baby for the first two months of her life. Just like Dr. Spock states in his newborn manuals, the colic does go away (eventually). And thank goodness for selective amnesia: If I had remembered the severity of colic with my first child or known the colicky course would be repeated with my second, I might never have decided to bear children again.

Colic in our family has been gone for many years now and my children have grown into gorgeous teenagers. My mother was right when she told me that colicky months make for easier teen years. My kids have been darn good teenagers up to this point.

But now I wait for the other shoe to drop. According to a recent study from the Journal of the American Medical Association (JAMA), there is an association between kids who had infantile colic and subsequent childhood and adolescent migraines. The most common cause of headaches in children, migraines are very difficult to diagnose and terribly uncomfortable for the patient. (It is important, however, to rule out other causes of headache such as trauma, infection or tumors).

Fortunately, there are some effective treatments for migraine, which is much more than can be said for the futile colic treatments available today. Is it possible we could treat colic with similar therapies used for migraines? Further studies are needed and hope is in our future. Perhaps the "colic curse" will be treatable for future generations of my family and yours. Who knows, it could result in expanded family numbers! ☛

CONSTITUTIONAL LESSONS FROM MY DOG APPLIED TO YOUR DAILY CONSTITUTION

My dog pooped out on me. No, I don't mean that my favorite pooch, Jett, tired too early on our daily walk. I mean she literally "pooped" on the sidewalk in front of the president of our neighborhood homeowner's association! For the nine years of her short life, she has never urinated or defecated during our one-two mile daily walk. Generally, she has more sophistication and reserves her daily constitution (as my British grandmother Mumsie called it) until we arrive home from our routine exercise.

Why is she now having bowel movement issues at 9 years of age? Well, I estimate she is 63 in human years (based on unscientific calculations) and is developing fecal urgency. Is the sudden urge to defecate normal for an aging canine? Is fecal urgency to be expected as humans age? Can I write a blog based on my dog's experience with #2? I must be running out of blog subjects.

Readers, before reading further, read this:

1. If this discussion of the daily #2 offends you, please stop reading immediately.
2. Discussions like these are routine dinner table subjects in my house. Aren't you glad your mother is not a doctor?
3. Is fecal urgency (the sudden urge to have a bowel movement) a precursor to fecal incontinence (inability to control the release of stool)?

The answer to number three is yes. In a portion of the population, fecal urgency could later develop into a condition known in humans as geriatric (older age) fecal (stool) incontinence (lack of control).

In elderly patients, geriatric fecal incontinence may become a social stigma, and many times it is a "don't ask, don't tell" problem. Doctors do not ask about it, and patients are too embarrassed to discuss it. The prevalence of fecal incontinence is about 7 percent among people over age 65, according to American College of Gastroenterology.

There are two main causes of fecal incontinence:

1. Fecal impaction, which is severe constipation causing blockage of the colon. Only the watery stool is able to pass the area of impaction, causing uncontrollable leakage of liquid stool through the rectum. For people with fecal impaction, it is important for a doctor to rule out cancer as a source of the problem.

2. Rectosphincter dysfunction, a condition most common to diabetics, as elevated blood sugars can damage nerves of the rectum. Biofeedback is the first line of treatment and can be very effective.

If you have any of these medical problems, I hope you will discuss them with your physician. Untreated, fecal impaction and rectosphincter dysfunction can lead to significant morbidity, depression and social isolation. Additionally, properly managing underlying physical disorders can significantly improve your ability to control bodily functions.

For the record, my dog Jett does not have cancer and she does not have diabetes. She is just getting older and I have to pay more attention to her bowel movements and bring my pooper-scooper bag on walks.

As Mumsie used to say, "A good daily constitution is a measure of good health." Therefore, I hope the best for you and your daily constitution! ☜

WALK, DON'T RUN. IT'S THE DISTANCE THAT COUNTS

My neighbors know that I love to walk my dogs. You can't miss the sight of me with two large animals energetically walking the streets of my neighborhood. While it is not easy to be dragged by two standard poodles at the same time, I find it invigorating to be outside and love to see my dogs sharing in the excitement of the outdoors. Running is out of the question. Because of prior surgeries, I have had to exchange the running shoes for walking shoes and have switched to longer workout times in order to get the heart-healthy benefits of this low-impact activity.

Now I can be reassured that my two-mile walks net the same health benefits as my fast-running younger child, who goes the same distance in half my time. According to a study in Arteriosclerosis, Thrombosis, and Vascular Biology, runners and walkers receive similar reductions in risks for hypertension, high cholesterol and diabetes. Even though walkers take longer to cover the same distance, they can still turn out as healthy as runners and even share the same risk-reduction for heart disease.

Here are some highlights:

1. The study involved approximately 33,000 runners and 15,000 (moderately paced) walkers.

2. Running reduced the risk for high blood pressure 4.2 percent in runners and 7.2 percent in walkers.

3. Running reduced first-time high cholesterol 4.3 percent in runners and 7 percent in walkers.

4. Running and walking reduced the risk for diabetes (first-time diagnosis) by about 12 percent.

5. Runners experienced a 4.5 percent decrease in heart disease and walkers decreased their heart disease by 9.3 percent.

What is the bottom line?

You do not have to overexert yourself in order to improve your health. Walking offers many of the same benefits without the harsh high-impact activity needed with running. Who knows? You could be even healthier than that guy jogging in front of you. Get outside, walk at a moderate pace, and spend a longer time enjoying the sunshine. Consider my option and take your dogs. They will keep you walking faster, and chances are they will also enjoy your same health benefits. ☛

PEPPERS ARE A NEW HOT TOPIC IN THE PREVENTION OF PARKINSON'S DISEASE

My husband sweats when he eats hot peppers. He told me the other day, "Anything that burns so much going down the throat MUST be good for you." I could not agree more. Peppers and similar vegetables contain nicotine (yes, like tobacco), which may decrease the risk of developing Parkinson's disease. It's a hot topic in the medical community: a 2013 Annals of Neurology article strengthened the association between the lower incidence of Parkinson's disease and the consumption of nicotine-rich vegetables, especially peppers.

Parkinson's disease is a nervous system disorder characterized by a resting tremor and slowed body movements. Normal gaited walking is replaced with shuffling of the feet, and balance may become more difficult, increasing the risk of falls. While Parkinson's disease normally affects the elderly, it has been seen in adults as young as 40. This study demonstrates the potential importance of healthy selective dietary intake on the development of this debilitating neurological disease.

While smokers have substantial risks for heart disease, stroke and cancers, it has long been known that their risks for Parkinson's are lower (presumably) due to elevated nicotine levels in tobacco. Foods such as peppers, from the Solanaceae plant family, contain more nicotine than similar foods such as tomatoes and potatoes. While regularly drinking tomato juice and eating baked potatoes have some protection against Parkinson's disease, the benefit was more closely tied to eating significant amounts of peppers (according to the study).

How many peppers a day to keep the doctor away has yet to be determined. But next time you order your salsa, request "extra spicy." You may breathe fire for a few minutes, but the benefits could last a lifetime. ☛

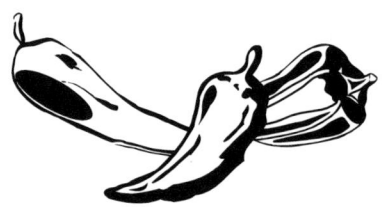

EXERCISE TO GAIN 'GOOD' FAT AND RAISE YOUR METABOLISM

Doctor, I may not be losing pounds, but I am losing "inches."

You cannot turn fat into muscle, but could you turn white fat into fuel-burning brown fat? The correct information is that your subcutaneous fat may be changing from yellow (white) fat to brown fat, accounting for improved body sculpting with exercise. So, maybe you are not losing pounds with exercise, but you are losing inches. Exercise not only improves muscle tone, but it may also change body-fat composition, giving you a more lean and fit appearance to show off your workout efforts.

Many years ago, physicians and researchers assumed that brown fat was only active in babies and children. Its elevated calorie-burning properties were thought to help children maintain lower body-fat percentages. Brown fat was thought to disappear as children matured.

But according to a study presented at the American Diabetes Association (ADA) conference in Chicago, exercise may transform unwanted ugly fat to more appealing brown fat. The ADA announcement reported the development of brown fat in men after 12 weeks of regular bike training.

Studies also found that brown fat is associated with improved insulin sensitivity and serum glucose levels in mice. That means regular exercise and transition of white fat to brown fat would lessen the risk for developing diabetes. Best of all, brown fat may burn fuel (more fuel points to gain on my Nike FuelBand!).

FEEL SUPER ABOUT YOUR STATIN SAFETY

I suppose I never get tired of blogging about statin drug safety, as I never stop counseling patients about statin drug safety. This morning, I have even more to blog about statin drug safety (have I emphasized "safety" enough times yet?).

Statin drugs are commonly prescribed medicines that when used daily significantly decrease the risk of heart attack and stroke by lowering "bad" (LDL) cholesterol in the blood stream. Statins also decrease inflammation in the arteries, and stabilize and reduce arterial wall plaque formation.

In Circulation: Cardiovascular Quality and Outcomes (July 2013), 135 previous studies, which included 250,000 people taking statin drugs such as atorvastatin (Lipitor), simvastatin and pravastatin, were analyzed. The extensive review concluded that side effects of statin drugs were very low and that the benefits of these medicines greatly outweighed their risks.

Though rare, side effects such as muscle breakdown and kidney damage (rhabdomyolysis) may be a cause of death. However, only 0.15 persons per million prescriptions experienced these side effects. While side effects of statins such as muscle pain may go up with the milligram dosage, lowering the dosage can help to avoid adverse symptoms and still allow many of the statin benefits. In addition, liver enzyme elevations that are rarely associated with medication use are reversible and have no long-lasting health effects.

Understandably, some patients are hesitant to begin statin therapy. While there is up to a 9 percent increased risk of developing diabetes associated with statin drug use, the significant lowering of cardiovascular complications (stroke/heart attack) is much greater. Researchers from the Circulation study reaffirm that the benefits of statins outweigh the risks.

Of all the statin drugs, simvastatin and pravastatin had the best safety profiles. I suspect that in a few years these drugs (in lower doses) may go over the counter. If so, I will be the first in line because while my cholesterol is normal, a statin "supplement" could still substantially lower my risk for heart disease. Heart disease is the number one killer in women and more prevalent than all the combined cancer risks. So, if statins can take me out of those morbid statistics, I am all for it!

Ultimately, the decision for statin therapy use involves a conversation with your doctor. While healthy lifestyle choices can improve cholesterol, most individuals with hypercholesterolemia (high cholesterol) have inherited it from their parents and require medical intervention to lower cholesterol to goal levels. So don't feel guilty if your exercise, weight loss and improved diet do not positively affect your cholesterol values. I know of several skinny vegans with high cholesterol, and it is not their fault! ☛

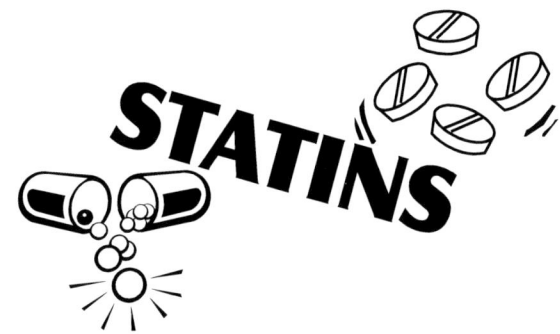

IS LACK OF ESTROGEN KILLING YOU?

I can hardly keep up. One day we are telling patients to stop estrogen therapy because of health concerns and the next day we are endorsing estrogen therapy for heart health. I understand how confusing it must be for women as they reach post-menopausal status.

Recently the American Journal of Public Health published an article that reviewed a 10-year history of "estrogen avoidance" in post-menopausal women. The Yale University School of Medicine's departments of Obstetrics and Gynecology and of Psychiatry devised a formula that found an excess mortality among "hysterectomized" (surgical removal of the uterus) women ages 50 to 59. Over the 10-year study, prescribed estrogen use had declined (between 2002 and 2011).

Over the 10 years, the study concluded, a "minimum of 18,601 and as many as 96,610 may have died prematurely due to avoidance of estrogen therapy."

As a physician, the best way for me to apply this information is to strongly reconsider prescribing estrogen replacement therapy in younger post-menopausal women (ages 50-59). But this study refers only to women who do not have a uterus.

The problem with post-menopausal women with a uterus is that a combination therapy with progesterone is needed to balance the uterus lining. Estrogen unopposed (by itself) in these women will lead to thickening of the uterine lining and stimulate bleeding, which could promote precancerous uterine conditions. When progesterone is added, it stabilizes the lining of the uterus and decreases the chance of bleeding. Unfortunately, progesterone with estrogen may promote breast cancer, heart disease, stroke and blood clots, according to the Women's Health Initiative, 2002.

The benefit of estrogen may be in the timing of its use in the perimenopause period. Estrogen confers heart protection by inhibiting hardening of the arteries and promoting good blood flow. But by age 60, changes in blood vessel cells may compromise estrogen's ability to prevent heart disease. Therefore, the window of opportunity for estrogen is limited but important.

For women who have undergone a hysterectomy, this study is reassuring for limited use of estrogen. Beyond age 60 the need for estrogen should be discussed with your doctor.

As a physician, I apologize for the complexity and confusion regarding hormone therapy for women. For years we have gone back and forth in our recommendations for or against estrogen replacement therapy. I hope this study helps put to rest our medical decision-making.

5 THINGS DOCTORS MAY NOT TELL YOU

Really, this information is not a secret. What you decide to discuss with your physician is highly important, and sometimes physicians, in an effort to run through your "list" of personal medical issues, will run out of time to remind you about basic medical advice or instruction that could significantly impact your health and/or your pocketbook.

Believe me, there are many more of these that I could write. But today I will list the first few that come to mind:

1. You need to exercise. Oh yes, you do. I realize you can't afford a monthly yoga class, but Denise Austin has some really great beginner yoga tapes. While the highly vigorous and physically complex P90X is not recommended for the average couch potato, many other exercise DVD options are available; you do not have to join a gym. If you prefer to walk, then WALK. Refer to my prior blog about lowering your exercise intensity, page 50. According to the American Heart Association, exercise can lower the risk for heart disease by up to 40 percent. There is a similar cancer reduction seen with moderate exercise. I always giggle when I hear patients repetitively tell me at their annual physical that they have "just joined a gym" (what a timing coincidence).

2. You need to lose weight. Calculations are that about 70 percent of patients in family practice offices are overweight. Doctors can easily become "burned out" unsuccessfully trying to get their patients to achieve normal weights. If your doctor is overweight, it is less likely you will have a discussion about weight loss.

3. Your medicine may offer a cheaper generic alternative. I will be perpetually grateful

for Wal-Mart's price-cutting initiative with generic drugs. The company's $4 drug list has come to the aid of many penny-pinching patients and allowed our Hope Clinic patients improved access to life-saving medications. While not all drugs have equivalent generic alternatives, many patients are able to reduce spending on most of their medications. Reduction of costs for a single medication can be several hundred dollars a month. For example, one class of blood pressure medications costs over $120 per month versus a $4 comparable alternative. Yesterday, a patient called to inform me that her prescribed muscle relaxant cost $175. I was able to offer her a reasonable $4 alternative. In fact, I raised the dose of the muscle relaxer, and the higher dose of the same medicine was cheaper than the branded lower dose medicine (so we broke it in half). If your drug costs are exorbitant, I recommend you pursue cheaper medication alternatives with your doctor.

4. You may want to reconsider some of your supplements. It is not unusual for a patient to come into the clinic with a long list of over-the-counter supplements. It is important to realize that supplements are not FDA-regulated and therefore may not contain the concentration of ingredients listed on the bottle or, worse, may have contaminants. Some supplements could be dangerous. From the Archives of Internal Medicine (2011): "... based on existing evidence, we see little justification for the general and widespread use of dietary supplements unless there is a medical reason or deficiency of a particular nutrient." In addition, post-menopausal women on supplements were found to have decreased lifespans compared to women without supplements. Proceed with caution if you take supplements and are on prescription medication. Be sure to let your doctor know all your supplements so that potentially dangerous drug interactions can be identified.

5. You probably don't need an antibiotic for a cold. According to several studies, 90-98 percent of sinus infections are caused by viruses, which means that MOST sinus

infections do NOT need antibiotics. Overzealous use of antibiotics can lead to superbugs and drug resistance. In the future, the antibiotic you need for a real bacterial infection may NOT work as well to fight your infection because of drug resistance and overuse. Wait 7-10 days after respiratory symptoms begin BEFORE seeing your physician for a cold. My colleagues and I agree it is much easier to give a patient an antibiotic, then explain why he or she does not need an antibiotic. When you have a clinic full of waiting patients, it is difficult to spend the extra time trying to convince a patient to withhold antibiotic intervention, especially when the patient insists on an antibiotic. However, if you develop persistent fever, shortness of breath or chest pain, earlier intervention is warranted.

Oh yes, there are many things a doctor could tell you in the exam room if time allowed. I have listed just a few of them. Most importantly, come to your office visit prepared with a list of questions, and be sure your doctor knows about all your medications (including supplements). Avoid taking unnecessary prescription (antibiotics) and nonprescription pills unless absolutely necessary. Engage and interact in your health care. We physicians care all about YOU. ☛

LABOR INDUCTION MAY BE LINKED TO AUTISM

Pregnancy is never convenient. But knowing when and where you will deliver your bundle of joy can make the uncertainty that surrounds pregnancy more tolerable. While many women dive right into labor without any physical issues, some women experience medical complications that require induction (medication to speed delivery). For those women, induction is mandatory. Perhaps the baby's water broke early, or mom's blood pressure is too high, or the baby is too big to wait until the due date. During labor, mom's contractions may have been too weak or absent. In many cases, medication (Pitocin) to hurry up delivery can decrease the risk of complications to both baby and mom by bringing baby into the world before difficulties develop in the womb.

Now a study from the journal JAMA Pediatrics (August 2013) suggests that women undergoing induction may have an increased risk of bearing a child with autism. OK, that is a red flag. Time to read more about this study and try to get the information straightened out.

First, let's understand the definition of terms. Induction is the method of stimulating contractions before labor begins naturally. Augmentation refers to increasing the strength and frequency of uterine contractions.

Here is a brief summary of the study:

1. Moms who had both induced and augmented labor had a 23 percent greater risk of bearing a child with autism.

2. Male children who were both induced and augmented had a 35 percent greater risk

of autism. Males born to moms who were only augmented were found to have a 15 percent risk for autism.

3. Female children of moms who were augmented had an 18 percent risk of autism compared to a control group.

The comprehensive study involved 625,042 live births, and data was controlled to account for maternal age and adverse maternal health conditions. However, several factors were not included such as paternal age and maternal medications. Also, data on the degree of autism and its severity relative to degree of induction and augmentation were not studied.

As stated in the JAMA Pediatrics article, one in 88 children in the U.S. is diagnosed with autism spectrum disorder. We all want the best for our children, and we really need to re-think delivery options. I will be the first to admit that for my second child, induction and augmentation was a matter of "convenience." In family practice, I have discovered parents in similar situations. For some families, the timing of delivery has to be perfect because the obstetrician or the husband is going out of town. Sometimes moms want to schedule a time that is suitable for work or vacation schedules. ☛

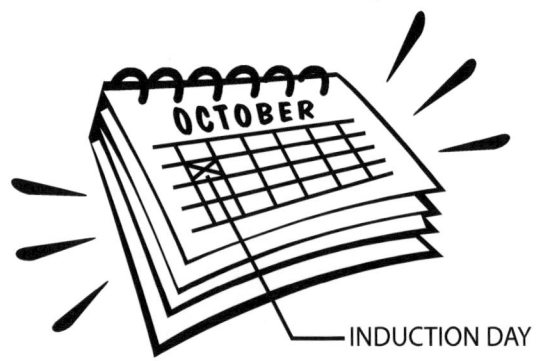

IT'S OK TO GO NUTS OVER COCONUT WATER

Rub it on, rub it in or take it in—coconuts are all the rage in the Dallas-Fort Worth Metroplex and are easily found in the refrigerators of well-supplied fitness clubs. But just because coconut water is popular, is it healthy?

While coconut oil has been used as a tanning accelerator (yes, I grew up in the '80s), its rich taste, high calories and high (more than 90 percent) saturated-fat content make it desirable in cooking as a substitute for animal or vegetable oil. Coconut water, on the other hand, is low in calories and both fat- and cholesterol-free. It contains electrolytes, including sodium and chloride, and (depending on the coconut species) may have as much potassium as four bananas. Coconut water is considered a more natural alternative to other marketed sports drinks and has even been used to rehydrate otherwise healthy adults and children with mild diarrhea.

Coconut water is the clear liquid inside young green coconuts. Coconut milk is the liquid that comes from the grated meat of a brown coconut. Coconut water contains approximately 46 calories per cup, and an 11-ounce flavored coconut water such as Zico, which some call "the ultimate hydration drink," costs you about 60 calories.

For regular and strenuous exercise lasting one-two hours, hydration with water is just fine. However, high intensity, time-extended exercise (triathlon/marathon training) benefits from electrolyte supplementation. We should recognize that coconut water hydration does cause abdominal bloating and discomfort in some athletes during training. Consequently, choosing between hydrating with a sports drink and coconut water is a personal choice. But no matter which solution is preferred, for most athletes, performance outcome will be equal.

POSTPARTUM PSYCHOSIS IS NOT THE BABY BLUES

The use of deadly force to kill a woman attempting to ram her car through White House barriers became live news coverage across the country last week. It quickly became obvious that the woman behind the wheel was acting maniacal and (most probably) suicidal. What was even more tragic was the discovery of her 1-year-old daughter in the back seat of the car.

We still do not know the reason behind Miriam Carey's bizarre actions except we could hypothesize she suffered from postpartum psychosis and/or other forms of psychological illness. According to the *Los Angeles Times*, medications for schizophrenia, psychosis and depression were found in her apartment. *NBC News* reported that she was out of touch with reality and felt that "Obama was stalking her."

With the birth of a baby comes a huge change in physical and environmental "structure." In fact, 70-80 percent of women will experience crying with sadness in the first two weeks following delivery. This condition, known as the baby blues, occurs in the first few days after delivery and lasts approximately two weeks.

While there are a multitude of reasons for feeling sad the first two weeks after the delivery of a baby, here are what I consider the three major changes contributing to the baby blues:

1. Hormone levels plummet quickly. During pregnancy, estrogen levels may be up to six times that of baseline, and experiencing a sudden drop to baseline levels can be quite unsettling for most women.

2. Sleep deprivation occurs. It is not just lack of sleep but also lack of one's own sleep schedule. The normal diurnal (morning-evening) sleep/awake cycle becomes completely messed up. I am certain this disrupts our cortisol "stress" hormones and contributes to mom's irritability and sadness the first two weeks after baby is born.

3. Focus of attention is on baby. The emphasis on "me" or "my husband" does an "about face," and all or most attention is given to baby and temporarily taken away from other family members. Therefore, fathers may also experience the baby blues (so, don't forget to shower attention on the new dad, too).

Postpartum depression lasts longer and symptoms are more severe than baby blues. Postpartum depression can begin anytime within the first year after childbirth. While women with a history of depression are at greater risk, up to 15-20 percent of mothers will develop postpartum depression. Symptoms include feeling blue, down, sad and tearful, with a lack of interest or excitement for upcoming celebratory events. A new mom might be sleepless or sleep too much and experience appetite changes.

Postpartum psychosis is rare, occurring in approximately one-two of 1,000 childbearing women within the first one-four weeks after delivery. Symptoms begin abruptly and are accompanied by confusion, delusional beliefs, mood swings and inability to normally function. These symptoms represent a major change from baseline mood changes.

I remember a case here in Dallas when a woman on the postpartum ward tried to use her IV metal stand to crash through a window so she could "get away" from someone chasing her. Another young mother tried to pump up a blood pressure cuff around her neck in order to choke herself. Luckily, both women were promptly treated and had close postpartum follow-up.

If you think you have postpartum depression, talk to your doctor and seek help as soon as possible. There are medical treatments that include antidepressants and counseling. If you suspect a family member or friend may have postpartum psychosis, please help her seek immediate treatment with a psychiatrist.

We really don't know if Miriam Carey had postpartum psychosis or if her postpartum status exacerbated some underlying psychological condition. But we can use this unfortunate experience as a wake-up call and learning tool to remind us that we must pay close attention to the emotional health of all postpartum women. ☛

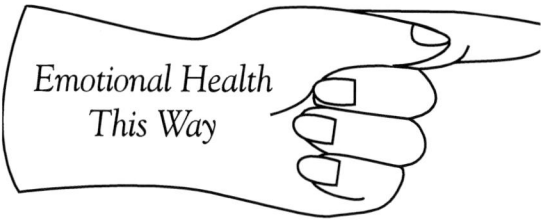

CELEBRATE STATINS! REDUCE DEMENTIA RISKS UP TO 3-FOLD

Running late, I rushed into the office and was greeted by an unusual expression from my nurse practitioner. "Is this a new look for you?" Heather asked. "Are you moving toward the dark side?"

What was she talking about? Well, in my rush to get to the office, I had accidentally pulled out my black eye-liner pencil and used it for a lip pencil. In the dark of my purse, they both look alike. But, oh my! I looked in the mirror and found myself looking like the old-time silent movie actresses who wore black lipstick (or a "vampire girl," according to my nurse practitioner).

When we are careless (like my example), we often wonder if we are "losing our mind." But really, for most of us, making a simple error is simply our inability to perfectly tackle our busy lives. Our minor mistakes are not due to lack of brain power.

I would, however, want to maintain excellent brain health as I age, and multiple times I have brought up the use of statin drugs as a means to avoid or delay dementia. Now I have more reason to celebrate statins!

A study from Amsterdam (yes, the Netherlands) found that people who received the highest doses of statin drugs (like Crestor, Lipitor and pravastatin and their generics) had a three-fold decrease in the risk of developing dementia.

The study is even more interesting because recently the U.S. Food and Drug Administration (FDA) listed statin-induced "cognitive" changes as a concern for the older population. This simple warning caused many of my patients to discontinue this vitally important heart-saving (and now brain-sparing) medication.

I should disclose, however, that there was evidence that a less commonly prescribed statin, lovastatin, at a higher dose was positively associated with dementia development. Lovastatin is a different type of statin (termed "lipophilic") and not considered comparable to other statins more commonly used. If you are on lovastatin, discuss with your physician if you could benefit from changing to a higher dose and higher potency statin drug.

Now, a question to my colleagues: Have I ever walked into a meeting with (accidental) black eye liner around my lips and you were too embarrassed to tell me? I am sure I have repeated this most embarrassing incident more than once. Perhaps, however, you should not tell me. I think knowing I made the mistake more than once could be harmful to an already suffering ego. ☛

LIVER FAILURE FROM A DIET SUPPLEMENT; BE CAREFUL.

A patient approached me this past week with a bottle of protein powder. He wanted to be certain it did not interact with any of his medications. The powder had a long list of ingredients, but to be honest, many of them weren't familiar to me based on my medical knowledge. I'd better do more homework!

As a former member of the Texas A&M Weight Lifting Club (yes, I used to be "buff" and have 6 percent body fat), I was obsessed with getting enough protein. Instead of processed plant proteins (powders), I preferred natural foods to supplement my diet. These foods included eggs, white meats and milk products. Ideas of synthesized or manufactured "whey" proteins or diet pills were foreign to both my peers and me. Actually, I was cautious of their contents, as protein powders and most diet pills have not been FDA approved and declared "safe" for human consumption.

Today, I remain guarded when it comes to protein powders, especially when the catastrophic problems facing people who took OxyELITE Pro seem to have confirmed my fears. Advertised as a "diet supplement" and "diet pill," OxyELITE Pro is presumed to have caused at least 29 cases of liver failure and hepatitis (acute liver inflammation).

While OxyELITE Pro was available in many states, the problems with liver failure all seemed to have occurred in Hawaii. The FDA had issued warnings against supplements containing dimethylamylamine (DMAA), which included OxyELITE Pro. Once the connection was made to this chemical and these tragic illnesses, the FDA issued a high alert. One person died as a result of liver failure.

Most people taking protein supplements will be fine. However, it is important to look for any DMAA content and stop the supplement immediately. Notify your doctor for any health concerns if you have taken this product. "Symptoms of (all types) of hepatitis include fever, fatigue, loss of appetite, nausea, vomiting, abdominal pain, dark urine, clay or gray colored bowel movements, joint pain, yellow eyes and jaundice," according to the FDA website.

While DMAA is highly concerning as a potentially lethal pill/supplement ingredient, most diet pills do not contain DMAA. However, there are other contaminants such as heavy metals that may be present in your diet pill or supplement. While searching online, I found a protein shake that contained significant levels of arsenic, cadmium and lead. One protein powder product had 16 micrograms (mcg) of arsenic, 5.3 mcg of cadmium and 13 mcg of lead.

How high is that? While many foods contain miniscule levels of lead and cadmium, according to the FDA, these lead and cadmium measurements are higher than the highest mean levels in a standard tuna can, which contains 0.32 mcg of lead and 0.02 mcg of cadmium.

A Consumer Reports article recently brought up concerns regarding high levels of arsenic in foods such as apple juice and rice. According to their studies, arsenic levels in rice ranged from 1.7-2.7 mcg per serving.

While rice, apple juice and tuna packaged in the U.S. are safe (for the most part), you can really appreciate (and be more aware of) the higher levels of metals contained in some health food supplements.

Be educated, careful and selective when it comes to your food and supplements. Go healthy and go natural! ☛

KNOW THE 8 SYMPTOMS OF DEPRESSION

In the past several months, our teams of medical providers have begun screening everyone for depression. Why? Because depression is a serious medical condition that is widespread and affects nearly one in 10 adults. Women are affected twice as often as men. Alarmingly, the U.S. Centers for Disease Control and Prevention (CDC) reports depression is present among one in 5 teenagers.

Blog-follower Vicki Anderson from the Granado Communications Group reminds me that October is National Mental Health Awareness Month.

Many of us experience times of depressed mood and sadness. But people with major depression (that requires some form of professional intervention) encounter prolonged periods of sadness that interfere significantly with their quality of life and can negatively impact their physical health. For example, psychological stress associated with depression can impact weight, insomnia and cortisol levels, thus increasing the risk for diabetes. In addition, having depression can increase your risk of death following a heart attack, according to studies cited by the CDC.

Now, grab a pen and sit down. Below is the Patient Health Questionnaire 8 (PHQ-8), which could indicate a diagnosis of major depressive disorder, according the Diagnostic and Statistical Manual of Mental Disorders, 4th Edition (DSM-IV). Circle any of the numbers below that pertain to your personal mood:

1. Do you have little interest or pleasure in doing things?

2. Are you feeling down, depressed or hopeless?

3. Do you have trouble falling asleep or staying asleep, or sleep too much?

4. Do you feel tired or have little energy?

5. Do you have poor appetite or have a problem overeating?

6. Do you feel bad about yourself or that you have been a failure or let yourself or your family down?

7. Do you have trouble concentrating on things such as reading the newspaper or watching television?

8. Do you move or speak so slowly that other people have noticed. Or the opposite: Are you so fidgety or restless that you move around a lot more than usual?

If you experience "more than half the days" of at least five of the eight criteria, you could have major depressive disorder. If you experience two, three or four of the eight criteria (especially including number 1 and/or number 2), then you may have another form of depression.

Please contact your primary care provider and get an appointment to review your answers in more detail. Treatment may involve medication and counseling (or counseling alone). But treatment is needed. If you lack personal funds, contact your local health department for access to counselors who can assist you. ☛

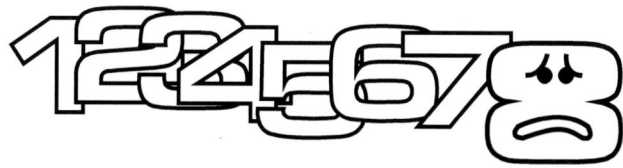

YOU DON'T HAVE TO LOOK OR SOUND LIKE DARTH VADER TO HAVE SLEEP APNEA

Reports of airline pilots falling asleep at the wheel have been in the news a lot. Pilot errors have brought to light the issue of pilot health and obesity and how it could impact passenger safety.

A few years ago, a flight to Hawaii overshot a landing strip by several miles because the two pilots had slept through their cockpit instructions and orders. *ABC News* reported that at least one of these drowsy pilots had been diagnosed with sleep apnea.

Sleep apnea is a chronic disorder associated with multiple breathing pauses or extremely shallow breaths during sleep. While respiratory pauses can last just three-10 seconds, severe cases may last many minutes. As in my most recent patient with sleep apnea, these episodes may occur up to 30 times per hour.

The repeated stress due to periods of oxygen deprivation leads to poor quality sleep. As you can imagine, low oxygen levels (over time) can stress the body, increasing the risk of heart attack, stroke, depression, obesity and diabetes. If you suffer from any of these medical conditions, you should speak with your physician to determine if you are a candidate for a sleep study.

While we generally think that a person with sleep apnea is a loud snorer, many people who don't snore also have sleep apnea. So you don't have to look like Darth Vader to have sleep apnea—you might actually look more like Sleeping Beauty.

While obesity is a common cause of obstructive sleep apnea (OSA), many lean people can also suffer from this disorder. Large tonsils and small airways coupled with poor sleeping positions can additionally lead to nighttime sleep disorders. Central sleep apnea (CSA) is not directly linked to obesity and occurs when the brain fails to send signals to muscles of the neck to relax. This interruption in natural air flow results in limited respiratory efforts during sleep and oxygen deprivation. Who knew that sleeping could be dangerous to your health?

Have an open discussion with your health care provider and get evaluated early before you experience complications of sleep apnea. Up to 80-90 percent of people with sleep apnea do not know they have the condition. If you have undiagnosed sleep apnea and wait too long to be evaluated and treated, you'd better have the "Force" on your side.

ACHOO syndrome is characterized by episodes of nearly uncontrolled sneezing brought on by sudden exposure to bright light from a period of relative darkness. It is a photic sneeze reflex and ACHOO is an acronym for **A**utosomal **D**ominant **C**ompelling **H**elio-**O**phthalmic **O**utburst.

DON'T STUFF YOURSELF AT THANKSGIVING DINNER

One thing I certainly give thanks for on Thanksgiving is the wonderful food. One of the best Thanksgiving cooks is my mom, who was born in England but who quickly learned how to make the most delicious cornbread stuffing and pecan pies.

I tell my patients to enjoy the turkey, stuffing, gravy, mashed potatoes and pumpkin pie, but with restraint. Eat less, eat slowly, and enjoy your food more!

Here are my three favorite ways to enjoy a skinnier Thanksgiving dinner (or any meal):

1. Drink water before sitting down to eat or approaching the buffet. According to Medical News Today, consuming two cups of water prior to your meal both decreased appetite and promoted weight loss. Water fills your stomach, which may decrease the release of certain hunger chemicals.

2. Limit or eliminate white and yellow foods. "Dr. Sadler, if it is white, I don't eat it," says my successful weight loss patient. Brilliant. Consider white/yellow foods such as bread, potatoes and stuffing as foods to eat in limited portions or eliminate all together. These foods tend to be the high carbohydrate, high fat foods that pack in concentrated calories.

3. Color your plate. Imagine a plate filled with green, yellow, orange and red foods. Color (according to the journal Nutrition) arouses certain feelings and sensations. Red seems to be highly stimulating for the brain and may even act as a "stop sign" for your stomach and reduce your appetite (according to the journal Appetite).

So on "turkey day" or any day, don't stuff yourself. Use these tips to save calories and enjoy a fulfilling feast. ☛

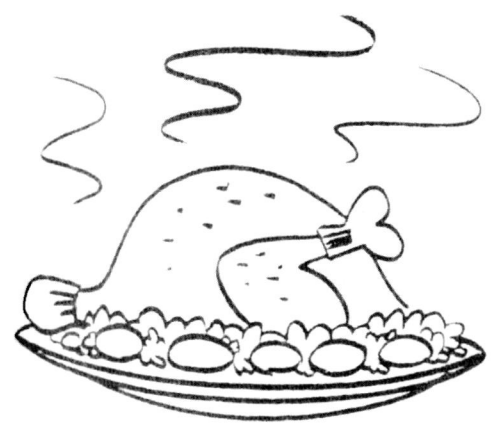

ARE YOUR REUSABLE GROCERY BAGS MAKING YOU SICK?

I have just finished washing my reusable grocery bags. So proud that I own them—I try my best to leave very little carbon footprint on our planet. I thought it would be easy just to grab them out of my car and go into the store, thereby avoiding flimsy, non-degradable plastic bags. But now my life just became more complicated: I have to wash the reusable bags.

Based on a recent study from Food Protection Trends, most reusable bags are contaminated with bacteria. The dreaded Escherichia coli (E. coli) was discovered in approximately 8 percent of bags, and large numbers of other bacteria were found in almost all bags studied across California and Arizona. Worse yet, if meat is stored in the car for two hours (who does that in Texas?), the number of bacteria increased ten-fold.

The good news is that hand or machine washing in warm water will reduce bacteria in the bag by about 99.9 percent. Just add bag washing to your weekly "to do" list (it is your list that grows daily). The benefits of clean bags are very good for better health.

YOUR KITCHEN SPONGE IS A GERM MAGNET

I hate throwing away a good sponge, but I have never really known how long to keep a used sponge or when to wash it (or how to wash it). For years, I have giggled at the frugality of a friend who regularly throws her sponge in the dishwasher to extend its longevity.

Why should I be concerned about the cleanliness of the very object that cleans my family's dishes? Perhaps because it is the same sponge I use to clean my dogs' feed bowls and countertops and sometimes spot-clean the floors.

According to a study in the journal Food Control (2007), contaminated kitchen items may account for an estimated 76,000,000 cases of foodborne illnesses annually in the U.S. Almost 90 percent of foodborne infections in developed countries originate from food prepared and consumed in the home.

But why point the finger at the "ever so useful" sponge? (It can't even defend itself.) Why should we give this small kitchen object so much credit for so much illness?

The sponge offers a warm, moist environment for bacteria and viruses. Some viruses such as norovirus (the leading cause of foodborne illness in the U.S.) can live in a sponge for up to seven days. Other common pathogens found in sponges include Salmonella, E. coli and Staphylococcus.

Studies published in Food Control demonstrate evidence that placing a dirty/contaminated sponge in the dishwasher for the full cycle or microwaving it for one minute at full power can decrease bacteria to near-undetectable levels. However, using 10 percent bleach, liquid dishwashing solution, lemon juice or de-ionized water were not successful in significantly reducing bacterial levels.

Bottom line: You CAN recycle your sponge. How often to wash the sponge depends on food contact and kitchen use, but I would suggest placing it in the dishwasher or microwaving it at least twice weekly, if not more.

Note to Sponge Bob Square Pants and members of his family: No sponges were harmed in the writing of this blog. ☛

SANTA, DON'T FALL ASLEEP IN YOUR SLEIGH

As we all sit by the fire this cold holiday season, I want each of you to spend extra time considering how to improve your health and the health of those you love. Maintaining a normal weight can prevent many obesity-related diseases including heart disease, diabetes and some cancers. Sleep apnea is a treatable condition that is linked to obesity and can be diagnosed and treated by sleep specialists. Consider a gift of a sleep study for you or your partner this holiday if you are at risk for sleep apnea.

Tomorrow the Dallas Morning News' Healthy Living section will feature an article on Santa and his annual physical. My concerns about Santa falling asleep at the sleigh are real. For my press conference on Santa's physical, see the YouTube video titled "Santa Claus declared 'fit for duty' at annual check-up." Here is my Christmas poem on Santa's annual physical exam. Hope you enjoy it.

SANTA'S ANNUAL PHYSICAL

'Twas the night before Christmas,
And all though Baylor Clinic,
Santa's name was being paged,
It was his Annual Visit!

His sleigh on the grass,
(Since a chimney we have not),

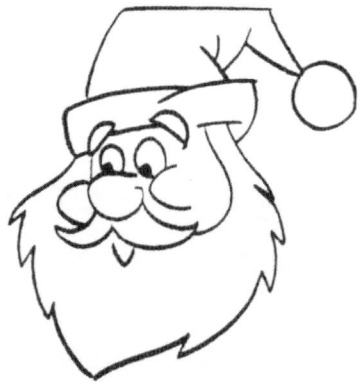

Rudolf grazing on the hollies,
Allowed to? He was not!

Santa was checking his list
When the medical assistant came in.
Old Jolly was still red-faced
And not all too thin.

Height, weight and blood pressure
The medical assistant reviewed.
Most above normal
(But we already knew...)

His weight and blood pressure
Were relayed to the Doctor.
The whole staff thought at once,
Santa'd best get off his rocker.

Heart, lungs, full skin check,
Head to toe they did go.
No allergy rash this year,
He'd been avoiding mistletoe!

Now off to the treadmill,
Stress testing HO HO!!
Run, run, run, Santa,
Now blow, blow and blow!

Full blood work, CXR
And that darned EKG,
Were standard for Santa,
(Risk factors, you see...)

Now the office again,
To talk with the Doc,
Old Jolly was nervous
He was usually a rock!

Secure login to update Santa's medical history,
Being HIPAA compliant to ensure his privacy.
Enter last flu shot, tetanus shot and colonoscopy
Adult preventative services save lives, you see.

"About you," said the Doctor,
Cholesterol high, sugars are stable.
EKG is just fine,
But push away from the table!

Get up from that chair,
Do not abuse it.
Take Rudolf for a long walk!
You KNOW he can use it!

Ease up on the cookies
And eat more good veggies.

If not, a chimney trip
Could earn you a wedgie!

And that fast food while flying,
May I make a suggestion?
Lay off the fries!
Learn to cook in the kitchen.

For one last suggestion,
Get out and play golf!
"Sounds good," said the Jolly Man.
"I will play a round with Rudolf!"

He turned in his chair,
Raised that finger to his nose.
Remembering what was just said,
Out of the chair he rose.

Out the front doors of the clinic
Saint Nick he did walk.
Proving to all
That he could walk the walk!

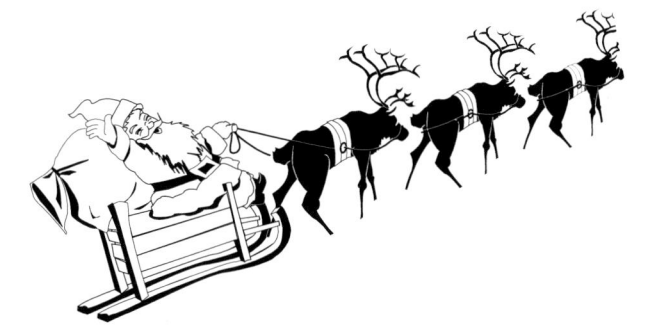

The sleigh then shot skyward,
All below gave great cheer.
And Santa boomed out, "Dallas,
I will see you next year!" ☞

DO YOU REALLY 'KNEE'D' SURGERY?

If you ask my husband, he would say yes, but a report on knee surgery in Finland (New England Journal of Medicine, December 2014) suggests that for many people, repair of a torn (medial) meniscus may be unnecessary.

Repair of the medial meniscus through a scope is one of the most common orthopedic procedures and, according to the study's authors, accounts for about $4 billion in U.S. medical costs annually. However, for many people, repair of a torn meniscus may not be necessary. In many cases surgery is the best option if conservative therapy fails. But this research reminds us that physicians and patients should discuss all treatment methods and their success rates before diving into surgery.

First, a simplified anatomy review: The knee's meniscus is the cushion between the femur (thigh bone) and the tibia and fibula (lower leg). The medial meniscus is the inside portion of the meniscus and is commonly injured in contact sports, especially when there's sudden squatting and twisting. In addition, degenerative changes (thinning) of the medial meniscus generally occur with age-related arthritis.

The study reported in the New England Journal of Medicine involved male subjects ages 35-65 with more than three months of pain. People with acute injuries and people with abnormal x-ray findings (consistent with arthritis) were excluded from the study.

It is interesting that in Finland, doctors were allowed to put all of the subjects under anesthesia and in half of them perform "sham surgery," allowing surgery incisions (cuts into the knee) without actual knee surgery. I doubt this level of study (putting all people to sleep and placing unnecessary surgical incisions) would be allowed in the U.S. (That is my blogger opinion.)

Nonetheless, after 12 months the average improvement in pain was similar for both the operated group and the "sham surgery" group.

According to Baylor Orthopedic and Sports Medicine specialist Dr. Anil Koganti, it was not clear if all study patients who had surgery had undergone conservative therapy or had other clinical evidence of arthritis prior to surgery. Dr. Koganti agrees that many surgeons and patients may be too quick to go under the knife, but there are many patients with acute medial meniscus trauma (excluded from the study) who could benefit from arthroscopic knee surgery. On the other hand, people with arthritis may not have significant x-ray findings and could have been included in this study. So it is not surprising that many study subjects did not find relief with surgery.

In general, Dr. Koganti recommends that patients with medial knee pain undergo conservative therapy that includes NSAIDS (anti-inflammatories such as ibuprofen), physical therapy and modified physical activity. In some cases, steroid injections into the affected knee can be helpful. For patients who have failed conservative therapy and who have significant pain at the site of the medial meniscus and show a tear on an MRI, surgery is certainly an option. For patients suffering pain due to arthritis and thinning of the meniscus, surgery is no guarantee for pain relief and has not been shown to delay or prevent progression of knee arthritis. Dr. Koganti has seen many such patients who refuse knee replacement, and removal of the torn meniscus fragment may be their only potentially successful treatment option.

Be aware that many orthopedic surgeons offer options other than surgery for your knee pain. Take advantage of their conservative opportunities before going under the knife. My husband's surgery to correct his medial meniscus tear has been highly successful, but the decision for surgery was made after almost a year of therapy. Some three years post-operatively, we are happy to report he is doing well and that in fact, he did "knee'd" surgery! ☞

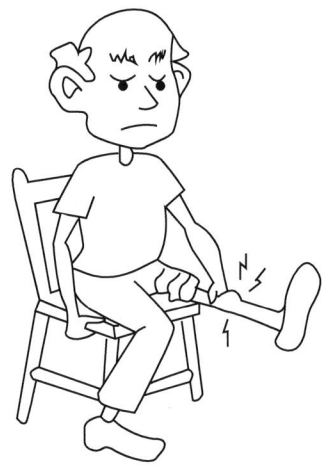

5 REASONS TO NOT BLOW OFF YOUR FLU SHOT

Make the relatively painless effort to get a flu shot because:

1. *You will g*et sick and could die. According to *CBS-D/FW* and the *Fort Worth Star-Telegram*, there have been 31 flu-related deaths in D/FW this season. Many years ago I was interviewed for Cosmopolitan magazine to discuss a young actress, Nicole DeHuff (movie: Meet the Parents), who died from complications of the flu. No one is "immune" to the influenza's deleterious effects!

2. You could harm someone else. If you get the flu and give it to someone you love (like your unprotected baby or grandbaby), it could be potentially disastrous. Treatment for newborns (less than 2 weeks of age) is not available, and all new moms and pregnant women should get the flu shot.

3. Without the flu shot, you could be at risk for a heart attack. People without the flu shot are up to 50 percent more likely to die from a heart attack. According to an article in the Journal of the American Medical Association (October 2013), people with high risk for heart disease benefit the most from the flu shot. Overall, everyone benefits from the vaccine with a lower risk for "major adverse cardiovascular events."

4. If you get the flu, you could miss several days of work (and that will cost you money). According to a Walgreens study, the flu caused up to 230 million missed work days and approximately $8.5 billion in lost wages during the 2012-13 flu season.

5. You have better things to do than stay in bed with a runny nose, aches and pains, a headache, a sore throat and a cough. Flu vaccine is still available. Contact your local health department, clinic or pharmacy to find out where to go to get a flu shot. Don't wait, VACCINATE! ☞

> Dr. Jane used to make fun of people who performed yoga and people who owned poodles. Nowadays, she loves yoga and her two standard poodles!

I VACUUMED MY DOG TODAY

When I got home today, my black poodle, Jett, looked yellow. Clothed in a sea of dry grass, she looked like a hay stack with legs. Tiny pieces of grass dropped off her as she walked across the room, reminding me of Pigpen, the dirty character in the Snoopy comic strip. The small grassy particles were stuck deep into her curly hair, so I did what any responsible dog owner would do. I reached for the hand-held vacuum.

Trying to keep my home clean and free of allergens has been difficult. My kids have allergies and, unfortunately, Dallas keeps their immune system busy with countless year-round allergens. To reduce coughing and sneezing, I have tried replacing air filters and keeping a clean house. We have replaced carpet with wood or tile and placed allergen covers over mattresses and pillows. Days like this, however, my efforts are futile.

But, all is well. When the allergies gets tough, the tough get going. We reach for the antihistamines. While diphenhydramine (Benadryl brand) may be the most potent of the allergy medications, it is the most sedating. In the last several years, prescription antihistamines such as loratadine (Claritin) and cetirizine (Zyrtec) have become available over the counter, and kids tolerate them well. Decongestants such as guaifenesin (Mucinex, for example) help to loosen secretions, while pseudoephedrine (found behind the counter with the pharmacist) will keep mucous membranes dry and nasal passages open.

When we first discovered our kids suffered from the Dallas environment, my husband insisted we have "low-allergen" (standard) poodles. But some days (like today), there is never enough medicine to counter "what the dog dragged in today." Thank goodness Jett loves the vacuum. ☛

REDUCING FEVER MAY PROLONG OR WORSEN FLU

As much as we try to interfere with Mother Nature, it is important to remember that the body has its own remarkably natural way of fighting infections. Most of the time, however, we prematurely reach into the medicine cabinet for relief of fever and discomfort. We feel that desperate times call for desperate measures, no?

"Pop" some acetaminophen or ibuprofen* and our symptoms temporarily subside. But what if the fever was intended to fight the infection?

A study published in Pharmacotherapy, (December 2000) compared the duration of illness in those who received anti-fever medication to those who did not take any drugs to lower temperature. The flu sufferers who took one of the anti-fever medications were sick an average of 3.5 days longer than whose who took nothing to lower fever.

Recently, an analysis was performed to estimate the expected number of U.S. influenza deaths directly attributable to fever reducers. In the Proceedings of the Royal Society B: Biological Sciences (January 2014) a study demonstrated a predictable increase in the death rate in the U.S. from the flu. It is estimated that 5 percent of flu deaths are attributed to the use of anti-pyretics (e.g., acetaminophen and ibuprofen). That action could account for between 700-2,000 additional deaths a year, depending on the flu strain that season.

Bottom line: If you (or your child) have a cold or flu associated with fever, let the temperature run a little higher. Temperature to 101 is acceptable and may not need to be treated. But if headache, nausea or vomiting are present and fever climbs over 102, then fever-reducers may be necessary. But this advice is not for everyone, especially if your child has a history of febrile seizures (seizures associated with high temperatures). On-line details from the Centers for Disease Control and Prevention (CDC) offers good advice on fever standards. It may be worth discussing your child's ideal temperature with your medical provider. ☛

*The medical professions recommend against the use of aspirin for flu or chicken pox (in children) because it could lead to Reye's syndrome, a potentially dangerous disease associated with brain and liver failure.

WHAT SHOULD YOU TAKE FOR THAT PESKY COLD?

An advanced medical degree does not shelter me from that "I am so overwhelmed" feeling when seeking cold-symptom relief in the supermarket's cold and flu aisle.

Oh, my goodness! There seem to be infinite choices of over-the-counter remedies for a variety of ailments, but research can help us wade through.

A journal article from the December American Family Physician nicely summarized studies approving some common treatments for cold symptoms. Surprisingly, many treatments that were reviewed could not be endorsed and should even be avoided when feeling ill. Other treatments work well, but may be associated with significant side effects, especially for people with underlying medical disorders. Antibiotics were found to be ineffective for treating symptoms of the common cold.

Let's look at what is in the OTC medicines. There are decongestants such as pseudoephedrine, phenylpropanolamine; mucolytics (designed to clear mucus) such as guaifenesin; antihistamines (which fight allergy symptoms) such as Benadryl and Claritin; cough suppressants such as dextromethorphan; and natural remedies such as vitamins and minerals.

Evidence-based data reaffirms that there is no single treatment that significantly improves common cold symptoms. Most of the OTC therapies combine some of the above categories to provide relief.

For instance, an antihistamine alone was not as effective as when combined with a decongestant (pseudoephedrine) for nasal congestion. Most medicines combined with pseudoephedrine work well to combat nasal congestion (Postgraduate Medicine, July 2008). A pill form may be equally effective to a medicated nasal spray decongestant (Journal of Family Practice, September 2003).

Not all decongestants are the same, even though their names may sound similar. The decongestant phenylephrine was found to be no more effective than a sugar pill, according to Annals of Allergy Asthma and Immunology (February 2009). However, the decongestant phenylpropanolamine was as effective as pseudoephedrine (American Journal of Rhinology, 2001). Pseudoephedrine sales are strictly controlled at pharmacies.

Mucolytics for cough include guaifenesin, which according to the National Institutes of Health website may improve drainage of mucous from the nose and thin secretions in a common cold. By loosening bronchial secretions, it could help to make coughs more productive. Guaifenesin may work better when combined with pseudoephedrine, according to Respiratory Care (2007).

Cough suppressants such as dextromethorphan HBR (Robitussin DM) are supposed to decrease cough frequency. Asthma patients should use cough suppressants with caution; inhalers are more suitable for managing their wheezing.

Relief-seeking can have complications. Nasal spray decongestants such as oxymetazoline (contained in Afrin nasal spray) are effective but should be limited to three days' use: Rebound nasal congestion can lead to physical dependence. Nasal saline sprays can help loosen secretions and can be used more often and for longer periods of time. Asthmatics should avoid combination therapy with aspirin; it could make their asthma worse. For cold symptoms, children should never have aspirin, especially in suspected cases of flu or chicken pox, because of potential liver damage.

Pseudoephedrine may increase blood pressure and heart rate and could harm patients with heart disease, diabetes, thyroid disorders and prostate problems.

Fever-reducing drugs such as acetaminophen and ibuprofen can make us feel more comfortable, but recent literature (out of McMaster University, Canada) suggests that suppressing fever for the flu may result in a 5 percent increase in the number of flu cases and deaths. An increase in body temperature helps naturally fight infection.

Natural remedies that have been found to help reduce the incidence and duration of cold symptoms include zinc lozenges (Cochrane Database of Systematic Reviews, 2013) and chicken noodle soup (American College of Chest Surgeons, October 2010). For nighttime relief, Breathe-Rite nasal strips work very well to keep nasal passages open.

Avoid zinc nose sprays, as they could cause nasal pain and damage your sense of smell. As popular as they are, echinacea and vitamin C have not been shown to help prevent catching a cold or to reduce subsequent symptoms.

In summary, if you are generally healthy, your immune system will naturally fight your infection, and your cough and nasal congestion should clear within 10 days. Careful OTC remedy selection can help to alleviate cold symptoms. Do not be shy about seeking advice from a pharmacist.

However, if your symptoms persist or they become more severe (including fever, shortness of breath or vomiting), you should see a medical provider immediately.

8 REASONS WHY ALL CALORIES ARE NOT THE SAME

"You are what you eat" are words you may live or die from based on your age and dietary protein intake. For years, the Atkins Diet has been the "go to" weight-loss method for millions of Americans hoping for quick results. Now, its methods are being called into question due to concerns about the health of high protein diets for people between the ages of 50 and 65.

A diet is considered high protein if caloric intake consists of greater than 20 percent protein.

Pay attention, because this is what you need to know. I get emails about the use of "natural" or synthesized protein/amino-acid supplements, but it is difficult to answer all of them. So, here is a synopsis of recent studies that, compiled together, tell a clearer story about high-protein benefits or possible health hazards:

1. People eating high protein diets and consuming similar caloric quantities may lose weight faster than people on regular or high carbohydrate diets, and diabetics' blood sugars may improve.

2. People age 50-65 on high protein diets may increase the likelihood of cancer or diabetes-related deaths four times over the next 18 years, according to a recent article in Cell Metabolism.

3. In the same age group (same study), high protein diets were shown to possibly increase the risk of dying of any cause two-fold over the next 18 years.

4. High protein intake may have detrimental effects on the kidneys (University of

Granada study, 2014)

5. The ill effects of a high protein diet were less (or possibly negligible) in people consuming diets high in plant-based proteins.

6. For people older than 65, the effect of a moderate to high protein diet was opposite compared to the middle-aged group. This older (my grandfather would instead say "wiser") group of individuals consuming moderate to high protein diets experienced a 60 percent decreased risk of dying of cancer and a 28 percent reduced rate of dying of other causes.

7. Amino acids (the building blocks of proteins) may decrease cancer-fighting properties of cells and increase damage to DNA. Therefore, high protein diets may increase the risk of cancer. (Does that make you want to reconsider protein "additives" in your smoothies?)

8. The ideal diet is the Mediterranean diet, which incorporates whole grains, low fat products, plant proteins, red wine, and fresh fruits and vegetables.

I LOVE EAU DE MOO! WHY DON'T YOU?

I love the smell of cow manure. My kids hate it. I suppose the odor of naturally processed grass does gross out a few people. When it is stuck on your shoe the experience may seem even far less appealing. For me, however, the odor conjures up nostalgic feelings of spending weekends at the family farm. Riding horses, running after cows and playing with goats and (more recently) a sheep make this city girl feel free to enjoy romping around in muddy, grungy shoes and to relish dirt on my hands and face.

According to Rachel S. Herz, psychologist at Brown University, a specific odor linked to a "conditioned stimulus" can bring about the emotional experience linked to that particular odor. Her theory certainly explains my joy of malodorous cow (and horse) manure. It also explains why a patient of mine complained about dreading the hospital and its sanitary "hospital smell" as a result of her decades-old Army hospital experience. To me, the smell of a clean hospital is a reminder of amazing patient encounters and friendly Baylor hospital staff.

According to Dr. Herz, hospital odors linked to surgical experiences may bring about "the conditioned response of anxiety when encountered in the future." Therefore, odors can elicit positive or negative emotions depending on the associated experience. I am certain (and hopeful) that the last decade of improved hospital quality and care have improved patient's "hospital odor" connection.

Not just between individuals, but also across countries, odors may be associated with significantly contrasting experiences. According to Scientific American (2002), in the mid-1960s, British adult volunteers found the smell of wintergreen in the "lowest pleasantness" ratings, while in the U.S. wintergreen received the "highest pleasantness rating." At that time, wintergreen flavoring was used in British medicine, while in the U.S. it was used for flavorful candy.

In my clinic, I place scented smells in some of the outlets. Interestingly, my nurse practitioner reported a happy feeling with the cinnamon smell but was not happy with the flower-scented oil. For me, the flower smell made me think of an unkind teacher from grade school and I did not like the scent either.

In the American Psychological Association (APA) journal (2011), research from Alan Hirsch, M.D., found that men might estimate the age and weight of females based on floral aroma. Volunteers who wore grapefruit scent were perceived to be 5 years younger than their actual age. Additionally, women wearing floral and spice perfume were judged to weigh about four pounds less compared to women wearing no perfume. If the men really liked the perfume and found it "pleasant," the women were perceived to be up to about 12 pounds lighter.

I know my boundaries and I am sure most people do not share my love for natural eau de cow. I think I will leave my joy for manure-scented oil essence alone for now and switch to a more youthful and lighter grapefruit and floral-scented perfume. Now it makes sense to change my scent. ☛

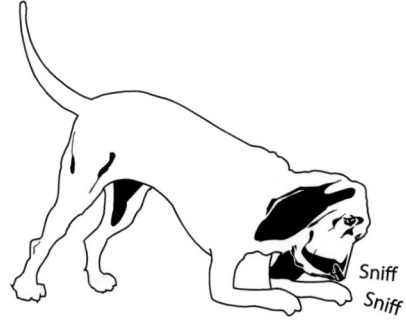

IS YOUR TEEN ADDICTED TO HIS OR HER PHONE?

In my clinic this week, I gently removed cellphones from the hands of several teens during their appointments. Distractions from video games and texting made it hard for us to communicate.

No less than four times this week I had to counsel teens on separating from their phones at night in order to get more sleep. My conclusion? Separating a teen from his or her cellphone is like separating a child from a parent.

I suspect that many teens suffer from nomophobia, which is the fear of being without mobile phone contact. According to the Indian Journal of Community Medicine (April 2010), some users develop "serious psychological dependence" on their cellphones.

As a parent, you must break the habit early and use interventional practices with your teen such as placing the phone outside the bedroom and silencing it at bedtime. (My husband regularly says, "Nothing good happens after 10 o'clock at night," and that includes cellphone activity.)

Other reasons to separate your teens from their phones at night come from research presented at the 22nd annual meeting of the Associated Professional Sleep Societies. It was found that teens who have excessive cellphone use are more prone to "interrupted sleep, restlessness, stress and fatigue."

In their studies, researchers chose 21 teens ages 14 to 20 with regular wake-sleep hours along with normal schoolwork and activities. Excessive phone users were those who made more than 15 calls and/or 15 texts daily, compared with the control group, which made fewer than five phone calls and/or texts daily. Some of the heavier users sent more than 30 text messages a day, and one sent more than 200 texts a day. (This was back in 2008.)

Compared to the control group, the teens with excessive cellphone use were more likely to awaken during the night and have more restless and disruptive sleep. They drank more caffeinated soft drinks and were more likely to consume alcohol. On the weekends, seven out of 11 heavy cellphone users slept until noon, compared with only two of 10 in the control group.

I will confess that both my teens send more than 15 texts daily, and I fear they often suffer disruptive sleep cycles. However, I insist on separating them from the phone at night. My kids think it is a joke that they need eight to nine hours of sleep every night. After-school activities and homework keep them up into the late hours. They insist that communicating with friends online and through texts improves their homework comprehension and maintains their healthy social network.

I am not buying it. More than just calls and texts, it is the push notifications, Facebook, Twitter, etc., that continue to impair their focus throughout the day and night.

In my era (we are going back to the '80s), it was television and telephone addiction. However, with five kids in my family, one phone line and no cable TV, our access to electronics was as limited as the wait time to our only bathroom was long.

Many years ago, I was interviewed for a TV segment on TTT (teenage texting tendonitis). I had pegged the term TTT based on my clinical observations of overworked thumbs and fingers on quick-fire teen texting and poor joint health. Now, my concern extends to the consequences of poor sleep associated with overworked teen texting.

The American Academy of Sleep Medicine has advice for improving teen sleep habits: follow consistent bedtime routines, avoid staying up all night to study for exams, cut back on after-school activities that interfere with study time, and keep computers and TVs out of the bedroom. On weekends, getting up at the same time daily (or even allowing an extra hour) also improves sleep hygiene.

Just knowing the ill effects of overextended teen texting time might lead some parents to consider tossing the phone out the window. It should encourage them to at least keep better oversight on the devices.

> National Puppy Day is March 21. This day is about bringing awareness to pet adoption (and loving on your puppies!). Remember, your puppies also need a gradual introduction to Texas heat before taking them on a long run. Also, have an extra carrier for their water bowl if you elect to take them outside for extended periods of time.

EXERCISE IS A YEAR-ROUND SPORT

It is a beautiful day outside and the weather is finally warmer! Time to reach into the back of the closet, grab the sneakers and start exercising again. What happened over the winter? There should be no dust on your sneakers; those sneakers are year-round style choices for your physical fitness wardrobe. Exercise is not weather-dependent.

In a few months, it will be "too hot to exercise." Unfortunately, Texas weather can be like a double-edged sword: too hot or too cold. The trick to staying healthy and maintaining regular physical activity is keeping flexibility in exercise choices. Choose sports that can be done inside or outside. Walking is easy because during cold, wintry weather or hot and humid days, the indoor treadmill can be your best friend. In addition, floor exercises, dancing, stretching and simple weight lifting can be done in the comfort of your own home.

Hot weather is just around the corner and your body may not be ready for the heat. Start your warm-weather activities with low intensity and adjust your intensity level as your exercise tolerance improves. Stay tuned to weather reports of high humidity because sweat does not evaporate well on those days and our bodies will not cool off as well.

Know the seven signs of heat exhaustion:

1. Heavy sweating

2. Headache

3. Nausea and vomiting

4. Fatigue

5. Dizziness

6. Muscle cramps

7. Cool, damp skin

Get going and good luck! ☛

> Approximately 63% of gym machines harbor rhinovirus germs. This bug is most commonly responsible for the common cold. Wash your hands well after a work out!
>
> *Clinical Journal of Sports Medicine*
> *January 2006*

$1,000 A MONTH ON SUPPLEMENTS

Kidney tests are declining, blood sugar is rising, and his chronic leukemia is worsening. "Bob" is on multiple prescription medications. Out-of-pocket medical expenses are increasing and his wife likes to go shopping. In addition, he is spending $1,000 monthly on nutritional supplements

I get it. More out-of-pocket expenses are incurred by patients than ever before. Benefits of prescription drugs are proven effective and approved by the Federal Drug Administration (FDA). But I have a difficult time justifying the high cost of his "natural" supplements, especially since the contents are unregulated and his recent blood tests are demonstrating declining health.

Bob assures me he feels "better" on the supplements and for now does not mind the high cost. The product supplier continues to reassure him that he will get better.

Multiple medical studies have come out to suggest that vitamin supplements can be more harmful than helpful. The Iowa Women's Study demonstrated an increased mortality in women taking (at least one) dietary supplements. In addition, the SELECT medical trial demonstrated an increased risk for prostate cancer in men taking vitamin E supplements. Cancer.org cites studies demonstrating an increased risk of lung cancer in people taking excess vitamin A. Even the regular use of a multivitamin has been called into question, and the Annals of Internal Medicine suggests it is a "waste of money."

People with proven vitamin deficiencies, however, do benefit from vitamin supplements.

Vitamin D supplements in people with vitamin D deficiency can decrease hip fractures, and iron may be necessary for patients with iron-deficiency anemia (until the source of blood loss is found and treated). B-12 deficiency (though rare) does exist. However, your medical care provider should follow these nutritional deficiencies closely, as over-treatment (vitamin toxicity) can be more harmful than the vitamin deficiency. Liver failure, vision changes, bone marrow problems and other problems can occur as a result of taking too many vitamins.

 My recommendation is this: Stop by Whole Foods, Central Market or Kroger's and instead spend your hard-earned money on fresh fruits, vegetables, and hormone-free chicken or wild-caught fish. Then, with all the extra money you saved from not buying supplements, send your wife out shopping. ☛

> A shout-out to the Fort Hood community and Baylor Scott & White for the excellent quality care they provided for our wounded Americans at Fort Hood. God bless all the medical workers and civilians who assisted in the safety, stabilization, transportation and medical care of our fellow Americans. Thank you, and may we all pray for an expedient emotional and physical recovery.

IS YOUR DIET SODA KILLING YOU?

I am always paying attention to medical news that most interests my patients, so when a patient asked, "Have you heard anything about diet sodas linked to premature death in women?" I sprung into action.

First, I was honest and told her that I had not read the American Academy of Cardiology's 2014 article, but that it was a perfect pending blog post. It was only a few years ago that I gave up diet sodas. During medical school, we would purchase 32-ounce Big Gulp diet sodas at the local 7-Eleven store. The high-volume caffeine content helped us burn the midnight oil, as late study nights were common. Luckily, my diet soda days are long gone. According to theheart.org, "older women (I'm not there yet!) who consume two or more diet sodas per day are 30 percent more likely to suffer a cardiovascular event and 50 percent more likely to die from related disease than women who rarely consume the drinks."

Researchers analyzed approximately 60,000 women ages 50-79 in the study. It was a careful study that accounted for weight, smoking, hormone use, physical activity, diabetes, high blood pressure and cholesterol among other demographics.

In the recent past, people argued that it was the artificial sweetener aspartame that put women at risk for premature death, but a study reported in July 2013 found that aspartame is not related to any significant (heart or cancer) health complications.

This is not the only warning for those with unhealthy soda relationships. My previous blog about sodas revealed that diet drinks could increase your risk of type 2 diabetes by as much as 20 percent. So here is my formal doctor advice: Drink more water (and tap water is just fine).

> According to the Journal of European Academy of Dermatology and Venereology 2010: Average fingernail growth rate was faster than that of toenails. There was no significant difference between right and left fingernail/toenail growth rates. The little fingernail grew slower than other fingernails and the great toenail grew faster than other toenails.

ARE ANTI-AGING HORMONES AGING YOU?

"Mike" arrived in the office looking super fit. The best I have ever seen him in the last 15 years. He was muscular and lean and appeared incredibly healthy. But he felt "terrible" and wanted me to take over the management of his care.

Mike has been seeing an anti-aging physician specialist outside of town and has been on a combination of three different hormone medications. But his medicine could kill him. Lab work demonstrated thickening of the blood, which could put him at risk for blood clots in the legs, lungs or even heart. For example, normal hemoglobin (blood concentration) is between 14 and 17, and his was over 19. His testosterone level was elevated beyond detectable lab values and his kidney function was on the decline.

Luckily, Mike was quick to be proactive and notify his specialist immediately for a dosing adjustment, and he has elected to wean off the medication under supervision and transfer back to our clinic for ongoing care.

Risks of multi-anabolic (muscle-enhancing) steroids include infertility, breast development, shrinking testicles, rage, aggression, mania, liver disease or tumors, stroke and heart attack. If users share needles, additional risks could include hepatitis and HIV. We know that exposing mice to six months of anabolic steroids significantly decreases lifespan.

As a young college student at Texas A&M, I was an active member of the Weight Lifting Club. Many of my friends were "juicing" with Dianabol (a muscle-enhancing steroid). Black-market suppliers were plentiful. I remember one friend injecting the steroid directly into his leg so that his "stork legs" would look stronger and match his large upper torso. (He reminded me of Mr. Incredible, the father star of Walt Disney's *The Incredibles*.) His legs still looked awkwardly small in comparison to his oversized chest musculature, and he became both physically and emotionally aggressive.

Despite warnings, anti-aging hormone therapy is a thriving enterprise. There must be a large number of people more interested in quality of life over quantity. I think Mike would disagree on the "quality," based on how poorly he feels right now. Yet, if there was responsibly managed and balanced multi-hormone therapy, would it be worth it to feel great for a few years in exchange for years of life potentially lost?

Unlike Mike, a few of my patients have been pleased with anti-aging hormone treatments prescribed by experienced physicians in the Metroplex. However, anti-aging medicine is an evolving specialty not yet recognized by mainstream medicine (such as the American Medical Association). Perhaps physicians are not listening to the needs of our patients and administering to their concerns. Perhaps there is a place for anti-aging hormones, although more research is needed to ensure patient protection, standardized treatment protocols and concentrated patient monitoring. The benefits must outweigh the risks. ☛

CAN THAT CUP OF JOE HELP YOU LOSE YOUR MUFFIN TOP?

Patients appear so embarrassed when they tell me the number of caffeinated drinks they consume daily. But actually, caffeinated beverages such as coffee contain natural antioxidants and can be healthy—but only if the coffee has no added sweeteners or cream and you are able to "stomach" its contents without heartburn issues.

The average daily intake of coffee in the U.S. is two cups (approximately 250 mg caffeine), according to Jon Ebbert, M.D., from FamilyPracticeNews.com (April 2014). Dr. Ebbert says studies have shown lower body weights in regular coffee drinkers. Most researchers claim that caffeine increases the release of natural body chemicals (neurotransmitters) that raise calorie-burning metabolism.

The journal Obesity (2013) published a study that evaluated the energy (calorie intake) consumed following ingestion of different amounts of caffeinated coffees. Both normal and overweight individuals participated in three trials. For each week, study participants consumed a breakfast along with 200 ml (almost 7 ounces) of one of three beverages:

Instant coffee with 3 mg of caffeine per kilogram of body weight ("Coffee 3")

Instant coffee with 6 mg of caffeine per kilogram of body weight ("Coffee 6")

Plain water

Three hours following beverage consumption, participants were offered a lunch buffet. The following day, they reported their appetite levels and total daily food intake. Interestingly, normal-weight individuals had similar food consumption (energy intake) in all three interventions (Coffee 3, 6 and water). However, overweight and obese individuals significantly reduced "energy intake" following Coffee 6 intervention compared to Coffee 3 and water.

The down side to this study? The average amount of caffeine consumed in the Coffee 6 group was 526 mg, which is equivalent to approximately four 8-ounce cups of coffee. According to researchers, the Coffee 6 was "not easily consumed by most of the volunteers."

Caffeine may be helpful in reducing appetite, but the dose of caffeine needed is quite tremendous and may be more harmful than helpful. High doses of caffeine can result in high blood pressure, elevated heart rate and heart rhythm abnormalities. These levels of caffeine can also promote irritation to the stomach lining, causing heartburn or even stomach ulcers. An even balance must be met in using caffeine for weight loss management, although perhaps caffeine could be one of many strategies included in your weight loss efforts. ☞

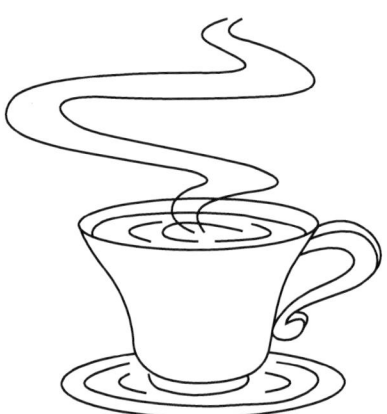

BEWARE OF BAMBOO BONFIRES AND RABID FERRET-BADGERS!

Most people do not scan the latest news from the Centers for Disease Control and Prevention (CDC), and medical literature may mean something different to non-medical people. No worries, I'm keeping everyone up to speed: The CDC has released warnings for people building bamboo bonfires (yes...bamboo bonfires).

Apparently 19 members of a family in Arkansas roasted hot dogs over a family-built bamboo bonfire. A week later, several family members became ill with stomach pain, vomiting and cough. Chest x-rays showed diffuse lung disease. Eventually all of the 19 relatives were ill with similar symptoms, and seven were hospitalized. The culprit? Histoplasmosis.

The Histoplasmosis outbreak was a result of bird and bat droppings (poop), which are a common source of the Histoplasmosis fungus (officially named: *Histoplasma capsulatum*).

The good news is that everyone recovered and has now been cautioned against burning bamboo, especially from groves where birds have roosted. Now YOU know.

Have you ever considered that rabies may not be a dog-specific problem? Also according to the CDC, Taiwan has discovered rabies among wild ferret-badgers (when is the last time you saw one of those?). Authorities tested hundreds of animals, and 31 percent of the 512 ferret-badgers tested positive for rabies. Ferrets are active at night (nocturnal), so (just in case) alert authorities immediately if you see a ferret-badger in the daylight because that probably means the animal is sick. For those of you traveling to Southeast Asia, please consider a rabies vaccination.

But why mention a rabies outbreak occurring in another country? Because rabies happens here in your back yard, too. According to local television station, WFAA, a rabies-infected skunk bit a young boy recently in Farmers Branch.

Rabies can cause serious medical problems leading to encephalitis (inflammation of the brain) and eventual death unless there is an early intervention. If you are traveling out of the country to a high-risk community, aim for prevention via immunization. Check out the traveler's website of CDC.gov for further information.

> Positive therapy-dog response today! Our Baylor therapy dog, "Happy," helped soothe a tearful toddler in the office. What a joy to have someone in pain leave with a smile.

WILL IT TAKE YOUNGER BLOOD TO MAKE YOUR BRAIN FEEL YOUTHFUL?

What if we could upgrade and recharge our brains just like we upgrade and recharge our cellphones? That would be great for older patients who complain that their memory recall suffers. Although I would love to offer treatment options for early memory loss or severe dementia, I have few successful prescription options at the present time. However, treatment to restore brain youth may be available in the future.

According to Stanford University, "blood taken from young mice may restore the mental capabilities in old mice." The study, originally published in Nature Medicine (May 2014), evaluated specific brain anatomy and physiology right down to molecular levels. According to one researcher, the results seem to reveal that some age-related impairments may not be permanent but indeed could be reversible.

Just like a working muscle, parts of the brain may enlarge when stimulated (exercised). An example in the article was a cab driver whose hippocampus (part of the brain) enlarged with driving experience. Further evaluation and comparison led researchers to report that the driver's hippocampus was more generous in size than the average person's. Interestingly, it is the hippocampus that is vulnerable to erosion with the aging process. This is the area of the brain where memories are made and stored. In people with Alzheimer's disease, the speed of hippocampal erosion is accelerated, resulting in their inability to retain and form new memories (according to the study's author).

When old mice received blood proteins (plasma) from young mice, the old mice experienced beneficial effects on brain (hippocampal) neurons. Scientists found that the treated old mice performed significantly better than untreated mice on learning and memory. The study has not yet been applied to humans, but some companies are already moving forward to begin human trial testing.

The bottom line: The old mice with young mice blood had more potential for learning and memory compared to their previous "old brain" function. Hmmm...perhaps Dracula had reason for choosing blood from younger victims—it kept his brain active! ☞

7 WAYS NOT TO TREAT A SNAKE BITE

Last week a teen patient came to a follow-up appointment for a snake bite. The unfortunate victim of three (yes, three) bites to the foot, "Drew" initially suffered severe neurotoxicity. The copperhead venom had caused a severe spasm of his back, with pain up his spine. In the emergency room, Poison Control along with his doctors elected to refrain from anti-venom therapy due to his rapid recovery during a few hours of observation. Unfortunately, Drew was not as lucky after his discharge from the emergency room.

Despite taking antibiotics to prevent a secondary bacterial infection from the bite, over the next 24 hours Drew developed foot swelling and increased pain. I saw him the following day in the office and immediately admitted him to Children's Medical Center, where he received excellent care and had a quick recovery with high-dose intravenous antibiotics. Today Drew feels "back to normal" and is even wearing shoes comfortably.

His is a story with a good ending. Yet if he had not had quick access to an emergency room and medical attention and hospitalization, he could have had a more tragic experience. Had the venom become more toxic to his nervous system, or his infection worse, he may have required surgery or long-term pain management. Luckily, he is young and healthy and was quick to recover.

With the warmer weather and wet days, many snakes have come out in the open to warm themselves. In my neighborhood, I almost walked into two large (non-venomous) snakes this past week. Be careful, especially if you live near a creek, lake or pond.

Most people know it is important to stay calm, remove tight clothing or jewelry around a bite, immobilize the area and get medical help right away. People should dial 911 immediately and try to have someone bring the (dead) snake to the medical emergency room for identification. Some medical kits contain venom-pump suction devices, but their effectiveness is controversial and most medical personnel do not recommend their use.

What do you NOT do for a snake bite? Here are seven tips from Medline Plus Medical Encyclopedia (with my comments in parentheses):

1. Do NOT allow the person to get too excited or overexert him or herself. Keep the person calm and, if necessary, carry the person to safety.

2. Do NOT apply a tourniquet (you heard me right).

3. Do NOT apply cold compresses to a snake bite.

4. Do NOT try to suck out the venom by mouth (unless you are John Wayne in True Grit, God rest his soul).

5. Do NOT cut into a snake bite with a knife or razor.

6. Do NOT give a snake-bite victim pain medications, stimulants or anything by mouth unless directed by a physician.

7. Do NOT raise the site of the bite above the person's heart. ☛

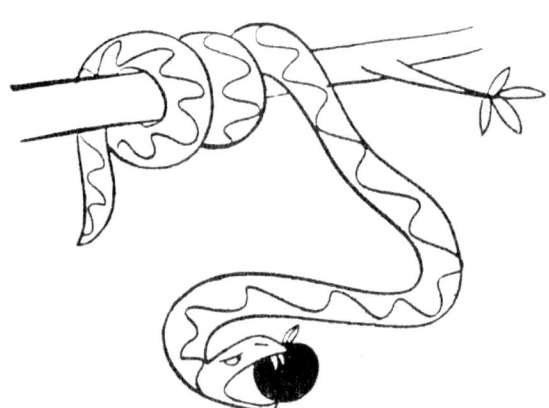

SHOULD YOU REALLY 'DRINK' TO GOOD SKIN HEALTH?

Why concern yourself with continually reapplying sunscreen in order to protect skin from potentially damaging solar rays? Why not drink to good health with a liquid skin product now available on the market? According to *Time* magazine, Osmosis Skin Care claims that its UV Neutralizer Harmonized Water protects you from up to 97 percent of harmful rays by using "cellular vibrations" and isolating "the precise frequencies needed to neutralize UVA and UVB" (damaging solar rays).

Just 2 milliliters with 2 ounces of water every four hours should be used while in the sun. According to the company, this repeated use could be equivalent to an SPF (sun protection factor) of 30. At the cost of $30, this product's 100ml bottle will last for up to 24 hours of sun exposure.

According to the American Academy of Dermatology, drinkable sunscreen is not recommended as an alternative to standard care and is not FDA (Food and Drug Administration) regulated. "The Academy continues to recommend that you still seek shade, wear sun-protective clothing and a wide-brimmed hat, and apply a broad-spectrum, water-resistant sunscreen with an SPF of 30 or higher," according to its website, SpotSkinCancer.org, a good source of information on sun protection.

It is interesting, however (though maybe not significant), that while sunscreen blocks up to 98 percent of UV rays, 2 percent can still potentially penetrate the skin and cause skin damage. Studies suggest that antioxidants such as green tea extract or polyphenols, found in tomatoes and berries, added to UVA/UVB protection may supplement skin protection. However, they are NO SUBSTITUTE for sunscreen lotion and creams. ☛

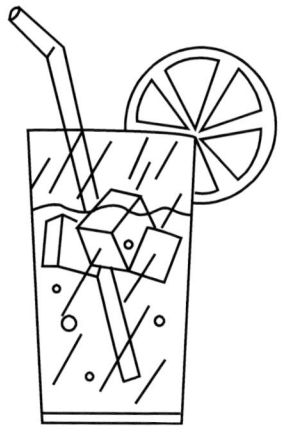

DO YOU 'KNEE-D' MORE MILK?

My mother received double (bilateral) knee replacements at the age of 72. At the time, her knees were "bone-on-bone," what we doctors refer to as severe osteoarthritis. The loss of soft tissue (meniscus and protective knee cartilage) in her knees had led to chronic pain, swelling and limited mobility. Undergoing successful surgery allowed her to continue to manage the family farm and live independently.

We look back (and look at ourselves) and wonder what we can we do to prevent the osteoarthritis my mother experienced. Glucosamine and chondroitin joint supplements have shown little promise in reducing joint pain and slowing the aging process. The recent American Academy of Orthopedics' Choosing Wisely campaign is now discouraging the use of these health supplements. For that reason, doctors have little to offer other than to encourage low- to moderate-impact activities, weight loss and injury prevention.

Now, however, we may have some encouraging news suggesting that milk is our knees' fountain of youth. According to the Osteoarthritis Initiative study (April 2014), drinking as few as seven (or fewer) glasses of milk weekly may be associated with less decline in knee joint space. In addition, the study said, "every increase of 10 glasses per week was associated with .06 mm less decline in joint space width over 48 months, compared with women who drank no milk."

Investigators followed 2,148 adults ages 45-79 with documented osteoarthritis (age-related arthritis) of the knee. Because some study participants had BOTH KNEES affected with arthritis, a total of 3,046 knees underwent annual x-rays and were analyzed over four years.

The study accounted for intake of other dairy products including cheese and yogurt, in addition to factors such as alcohol consumption, vitamin D intake, physical activity and obesity. The positive effect of milk (not other dairies) on joint health was found only among women (sorry guys).

While this study seems convincing enough for us to run to the store and pick up gallons of milk, I would caution that milk does have significant natural sugars and calories. However, milk is an excellent natural source of calcium and vitamin D (which many women lack).

Additionally, this study should encourage more studies to determine the SPECIFIC ELEMENT in milk that perhaps could be concentrated and provided as a convincing health supplement that potentially could prolong our knee longevity. Also, we need to find out why men did not receive the same health benefits from milk.

The bottom line for all you women: Looks like milk is important for "knee-d" health.

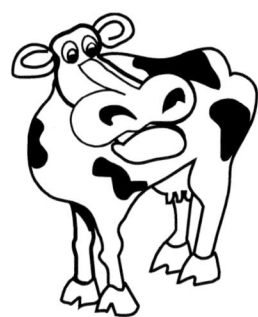

Have you ever seen a cow with bad knees?

I CUT MY FINGER AND FOUND 6 STEPS FOR MORE RAPID WOUND CARE

Yesterday, I cut my finger while cutting kale. It bled quite a bit, but luckily I sprung into action and was able to control the bleeding with a little pressure and wound-care glue. Unfortunately, keeping the wound covered became difficult in the clinic. I continued to wash my hands and diligently replaced my skin bandage in between every patient visit.

Within two days my wound was looking much better. I have to attribute the rapid healing to keeping the wound moist with antibiotic ointment and covering it with a bandage. But why not let it "air dry" or "leave it open and let it dry out," the way many patients have said they care for their own wounds? The answer is quick and simple: Moist wounds heal better and with less scarring than wounds allowed to stay dry and without coverage.

According to Medical News Today, the (European) medical community's consensus is that "rapid healing of the wound is best achieved by providing a moist environment." According to the medical data, a moist environment increases the rate of wound repair by approximately 40 percent. This is compared to leaving a wound to "dry out" and allowing a dry "scab" to form. Almost as enlightening, the article points out that moist wound healing reduces the risk for scarring.

I reviewed the information with the Baylor Garland Comprehensive Wound Center charge nurse Salma Sheikh, RN. She concurs with the information based on her extensive wound-care experience. With her help, we developed six steps to better wound-care healing for minor skin injuries (i.e., cuts and scrapes):

1. Immediately and gently clean the wound with soap and tap water, normal saline (if available) or distilled water.
2. Don't use peroxide or betadine, as these chemicals could potentially injure exposed wound tissue.
3. Place antibiotic salve on the wound and cover with a bandage. This will offer better protection from infection.
4. If the tissue around the wound turns white, there may be too much moisture. Change the dressing and create a better moisture balance.
5. Clean and change the bandage at least once or twice daily, unless otherwise directed by your medical provider.
6. If redness, warmth, swelling or increased pain occur, see a medical provider immediately. You may have developed a secondary infection and may need oral antibiotics.

Conclusion? Be careful when you are cutting kale (or anything for that matter), and have a great (and wound-free) summer! ☛

GODZILLA SPREADING SALMONELLA IN NEW YORK CITY

Is it just me, or does anyone else worry about Godzilla's slimy, bacterial-infested body raging through New York City? Sure, he is mowing down (empty) skyscrapers and other buildings, but he is leaving his amphibious germs throughout the city, too.

That oversized iguana is full of bacterial Salmonella. If people are not getting hurt from falling skyscrapers (which apparently they are not), they could certainly become seriously ill from his slimy residue.

But Godzilla-ravaged New Yorkers are not the only ones at risk for Salmonella infection. If you own or touch reptiles or amphibians, you are at risk as well. Most people associate Salmonella with contaminated foods, but many popular pets including turtles, frogs, iguanas, snakes and chameleons carry the illness.

People infected with Salmonella may experience diarrhea (often bloody), vomiting, fever and stomach pain. When people with low immunity develop Salmonella, the infection can spread to the bloodstream, causing serious organ inflammation or destruction. Antibiotic intervention is needed in those cases in order to prevent further organ damage or death. However, most people recover from Salmonella without medical intervention.

According to the Centers for Disease Control and Prevention (CDC), Salmonella affects approximately 1.2 million people annually, resulting in about 23,000 hospitalizations and 450 deaths. Of course this number could be higher if Godzilla decides to take over New York.

To avoid Salmonella infection, wash your hands with warm water and soap immediately after coming in contract with a reptile or amphibian. These animals tend to urinate when stressed, so be sure to wash your contaminated clothing, too.

Children under age 5, older adults and people with lower immunity (on chemotherapy or with HIV, for example) should avoid these animals altogether.

Be careful and protect the animal from your own germs as well. My sister's children have a beautiful bearded dragon and my sister correctly insists the kids wash their hands both before they play with it (to protect it from human bacteria) and after.

Well, I may be a nerd, but I enjoy watching the older versions of *Godzilla*. My son tells me the latest film release is "even better." I will eventually watch the new *Godzilla* movie, but I know that afterward I will feel the need to wash my hands.

Be selective and research local family doctors before choosing your primary care provider. Find a family doctor who is comprehensive, detailed, and performing a wide range of medical services. A high quality family doctor could reduce your risk of hospitalization by up to 35% and lessen your medical costs by 10-15%.
(Annals of Family Medicine, May/June 2015)

WHY YOU SHOULD BE 'THAT GIRL' (OR GUY)!

"Mom, don't be that girl that asks all the questions," was my daughter's reaction to my multitude of questions at our recent college tour. Well, I am sorry, but I will be "that girl" because I want to be informed and prepared to help her make excellent choices when it comes to her final college decision.

You should also be 'that girl' (or guy) when it comes to your medical office visit. Studies show that patients who are more engaged in their medical care have better health outcomes. According to these studies, benefits in self-care and lifestyle changes have been noted in conditions such as diabetes, coronary heart disease, heart failure and rheumatoid arthritis.

Too much information is overwhelming to many patients when it comes time to leave the office visit. While most clinics and hospitals provide printed handouts with instructions and a list of medication, the handouts usually end up in the trash. Let's face it, reading medical instructions can be like reading lines of Egyptian hieroglyphics—far too confusing, and the pictures don't help.

In our clinic, we highlight important elements in the patient instructions and, as often as possible, verbally review items before patients leave the office. Now we are able to post discharge instructions to our patients' private Internet sites. But, navigating the information can add to patient confusion and lead to possible lack of medical compliance, so sometimes we stick to a printable option.

Whether your personal medical advice is delivered by Internet, print, or pen and paper, be sure that the information is understandable. Shared medical decision-making (a little "push and pull") between you and your medical provider regarding medication versus adding healthier lifestyle choices can drastically change the direction of your care.

The trick is that we (your medical provider) make certain that medical instructions are as simple as possible (I know...I am working on it), and that we personally review needed medications and/or lifestyle changes with each patient. In addition, YOU must be "that girl" (or guy) and ASK questions if instructions are not clear. Help us to optimize a healthier you. ☛

YOUR DOCTOR MAY SEE A PROBLEM WITH YOUR CHILD'S WEIGHT

People say we have a difficult time looking at ourselves subjectively in the mirror. Most women, for example, view themselves as overweight, while only one in 17 view themselves as "slim." Accordingly, would we expect ourselves to be as critical in the way we look at our children's body types? The answer is no, according to a recent study. In fact, the answer is quite the opposite and the problem appears to be expanding (pardon the pun) over the years.

From a review of years 2005 through 2010, 83 percent of parents of an overweight boy and 78 percent of parents of an overweight girl considered their child "about the right weight." This is increased from the previous decade, when the percentages were approximately 5 percent and 15 percent lower, respectively.

Unfortunately, this misconception of child health can be awkward in the clinical setting. Many parents first appear shocked and upset that I would bring up concerns about their child's excessive weight. On the other hand, other parents seem relieved to break the ice and begin an open discussion about the need for improved weight management.

Fortunately, my data is objective and I am able to share graphs of the individual's growth in order to objectively demonstrate the child's weight category in percentiles. In addition, we can see trends over several years and estimate the trajectory of weight gain if the child were to continue on his or her same individual curve (or sometimes a straight upward line). When managed gently, these graphs can tell a story that opens doors to discussion on healthy nutrition and exercise.

Telling a child and a parent that there may be an issue with weight can be extremely uncomfortable if both are caught by surprise. Sometimes changing parental perception can be difficult, especially if the parent is overweight. Approximately 50 percent of obese children have obese parents, so changing to healthy lifestyles becomes far more complex as you work to manage household change.

Medical providers want to help you raise your kids in a way that encourages them to live long and healthy lives. However, parents must be willing to have someone else look in the mirror to more objectively manage and improve the health of their kids. ☛

> Trust your gut—if it is artificially sweet,
> it is probably artificially healthy.

WHAT DOES ELEVATED BLOOD SUGAR HAVE TO DO WITH CANCER?

I cannot help that I have a passion for Cheetos and dark chocolate! However, when my physician announced that my fasting glucose (blood sugar) was borderline elevated, I was appalled. Despite maintaining a normal weight and a regular exercise program, my love for carbohydrates and chocolate had proven to be my downfall. Thankfully, I am not diabetic, but I must be cautious due to a family history of diabetes. And, a recent study suggests my borderline blood sugar elevations not only might lead to diabetes, but could place me at higher risk for some cancers.

It is not uncommon to see mildly elevated blood sugars in people without diabetes. But subtle blood sugar elevations may signal a prediabetes condition that should be a knock on the door for lifestyle changes. According to the American Diabetes Association, a fasting blood sugar over 100 mg/dl is considered abnormal, and daily healthy choices must begin in order to avoid becoming diabetic.

In addition to well-known diabetes-related complications, there is even more reason to pay attention to your medical provider's advice when it comes to your elevated glucose (blood sugar). Elevated blood sugars could increase your risk of cancer by as much as 15 percent.

An article released in the journal Diabetologia (September 2014) analyzed approximately 900,000 participants from 16 different studies. Individuals with prediabetes were found to be at increased risk for liver, stomach and colorectal cancer.

The story is not just about losing weight, but about dropping blood sugar. Adjusting for weight (BMI), researchers found that the increased risk of cancer with prediabetes was independent of and therefore not associated with obesity.

A few years ago, the New England Journal of Medicine reviewed deaths associated with diabetes and discovered that affected individuals had increased risk for premature death from heart disease (stroke, heart attack, etc.). At the time, researchers also found associated increased risk for premature-death nonvascular (non-heart related) factors, including an increased risk for several cancers, infectious diseases, degenerative disorders and "intentional self-harm" (suicide).

The best way to avoid significant diabetic complications is to avoid getting diabetes altogether. I recommend yearly fasting blood sugars, cholesterol and symptom-directed studies as part of your annual physical exam. Especially with this latest information linking prediabetes and cancer, any elevations in your blood sugars should be seriously addressed and closely followed. Appropriate cancer screening studies should be reviewed with your health care provider.

For the last year or so, I have changed to "meatless Mondays" and transitioned to developing the flexitarian lifestyle along with a lower carbohydrate diet. This healthy form of living should help me to improve my blood sugar numbers as I move away from my much-loved Cheetos and dark chocolate diet.

To avoid prediabetes and diabetes, the American Diabetes Association can better direct you to healthier and (possibly) longer cancer-free living. Go to your clinic, get checked out, and pay attention to your blood sugar numbers.

ARTIFICIAL SWEETENERS: TRUST YOUR GUT

I had a "gut feeling" that artificial sweeteners could not be all that healthy. First of all, any food that includes the word "artificial" can't be that good for you; second, I have previously warned readers that artificial sweeteners are linked to obesity and its health complications.

Now there is direct evidence that artificial sweeteners may be as much a cause of type 2 diabetes as eating excessive sugar is. And it probably has a lot to do with changes in the gut bacteria (microbes) that help digest food. Researchers at Israel's Weizmann Institute of Science examined the link between intestinal bacteria and aspartame, sucralose and saccharine (all artificial sweeteners). Both in mice and in people, a transient two- to four-fold increase in blood sugars were found immediately after sweetener consumption.

Researchers found that people consuming the most artificial sweeteners had more problems controlling blood sugar and that mice fed saccharine had the most significant increases in blood sugar levels. So quantity of sweetener and type of sweetener both are independent risk factors for diabetes. The use of excessive saccharine probably is the worse (remember Tab soda...do they still make that drink?).

Additional studies were carried out on "bug-free" mice. These are mice that were developed to have NO intestinal bacteria. Interestingly (and quite gross), these bug-free mice were then fed feces of normal mice that had eaten artificial sweeteners (I hope you can "stomach" this). Consequently, these (previously) bug-free mice experienced blood sugar elevations after consuming artificial sweeteners.

Bottom line: Gut bacteria seemed to be responsible for the increases in blood sugar levels seen with artificial sweetener ingestion.

Other published studies have suggested gut bacteria play a role in obesity. For example, changes in gut bacteria in infants may promote early excessive weight gain. Multiple studies have linked weight gain to changes in gut bacteria.

If a man's heart is through his stomach, then we are all potentially healthier if we lay off the artificial sweeteners and have a change of heart when it comes to our diet soda intake. You are what you eat is so cliché, yet so true. ☛

The effective radiation dose from a chest X-ray is equivalent to 10 days of natural background radiation and carries minimal lifetime risk for fatal cancers. A chest computed tomography (CT) dose is equivalent to 2 years of natural background radiation and an abdominal and pelvic CT (combined with contrast material) is equivalent to 7 years of natural background radiation. Both CT scans increase the lifetime risk of fatal cancers.

American College of Radiation (ACR)

IS THERE A VIRUS INSIDE US? MOST LIKELY, YES!

While there may not be a fungus among us, we most probably harbor at least five different viruses. In a recent study published in the journal BMC Biology, approximately 92 percent of people have at least one virus. Are you thinking, "Not me!"? Think again. Researchers at Washington University in St. Louis sampled 102 healthy people between ages 18 and 40 and found at least one type of virus. In some cases, there were up to 10-15 different viruses in a sampling of up to five body sites per person, which included the nose, skin, mouth, vagina and stools.

Human papillomavirus (HPV) was found in about 75 percent of skin samples, 50 percent of nose samples and 38 percent of (female) vaginal samples. HPV has many different strains—some put women at increased risk of cervical cancer, and some have been increasingly responsible for promoting head and neck cancers in young men.

Several non-sexually transmitted viral infections were discovered. Herpes virus (oral herpes virus types) was detected among 98 percent of participants' mouth samples. Other viruses such as adenoviruses, which are commonly responsible for the common cold and more serious conditions such as pneumonia, were also found. Viruses were generally dormant (sleeping) and therefore not causing symptoms in the study's healthy population.

While the news may sound surprising, I don't find it especially shocking. Our body plays host to numerous bacterial species. We know that our noses normally shelter multiple bacteria including Staphylococcus and Streptococcus species. In addition, a woman's vaginal area will normally contain yeast and different species of bacteria. So why not add viruses to the party mix? It is thought that the perfect host environment is a balance of these bugs, which helps to maintain a normal immunity. It is only when one of these bugs grows out of control that we develop symptoms.

Chemicals and antibiotics can disrupt these environments and promote growth of yeast or cause diarrhea in some instances. Perhaps by changing our baseline body flora,* antibiotics could promote the activation of these sleeping viruses, making us more susceptible to illness

This new information is timely because as we approach fall, there is a rise in respiratory infection numbers. It is important to remember that most respiratory infections are viral and therefore don't need antibiotics, which can disrupt normal flora and perhaps worsen symptoms or delay recovery. Instead, let the body heal naturally in order to maintain its normal healthy flora. ☛

*Flora is defined here as microorganisms that normally occupy a particular body organ (such as the stomach or intestines).

5 SURPRISING HEALTH BENEFITS OF COFFEE

Just after my mother was admitted to the hospital for heart-beat irregularities, all her children came to visit. In a family of three doctors and two lawyers, I was the first to pipe up and ask my mother if I could run out and buy her a most coveted drink. "Coffee!" my cardiologist sister blurted out, "but she is in the hospital for heart palpitations!" OK...in my best efforts to provide comfort food and drink to my mother, clearly I was not thinking like a doctor.

But for most of you, go ahead, have another cup of joe. That cup of coffee (minus the sugar and cream) may be the natural health supplement your body needs. This is interesting and important for health care providers because our health-screening questionnaire includes the question "How many cups of coffee do you drink daily?" Historically, this portion of the questionnaire suggests that high coffee consumption is risky business. But now evidence shows that you may keep enjoying your coffee and its health benefits, and here are five reasons why:

1. Drinking three-five cups of coffee a day significantly reduces the risk for heart disease and stroke. Funny, in medicine we have always encouraged our high-risk patients to avoid or significantly reduce their caffeine intake. Forgive me...my brain is re-processing all this information, but "responsible" daily consumption of coffee (two-three 6-ounce cups) may have positive heart-health benefits. Interestingly, drinking much higher levels of coffee was not associated with an increase in either stroke or heart attack.

2. Coffee may reduce the risk of cancer. Regular coffee drinking may reduce the risk of

death from cancer. But don't only chalk it up to the caffeine; polyphenols and other "heterocyclic substances" in coffee also have benefits. Specifically, evidence suggests that regular coffee consumption is associated with reduced risk for liver, kidney and bladder cancer. To a "lesser extent," regular coffee intake may decrease the incidence of early onset breast cancer and colorectal cancers.

3. Caffeine may reduce the risk of developing Alzheimer's disease. According to the journal Neurobiology of Aging, studies demonstrate that caffeine reduces activity against particular chemicals that promote brain plaques. These amyloid deposits have a contributory role in Alzheimer's. Up to three cups of coffee a day may be protective.

4. Caffeine may protect liver health. The Brazilian Journal of Infectious Disease along with the Annals of Epidemiology report that consuming caffeine (more than 123 mg/day) was associated with reduced liver inflammation and scarring.

5. Coffee may reduce the risk for Parkinson's disease. According to the Centers for Disease Control and Prevention (CDC), with moderate coffee consumption, Parkinson's may be reduced by as much 25 percent.

Overall, the positives are strong for your daily cup of black coffee. However, if you are ordering a grande (more than 6 ounces), adding the half-and-half, doubling up on the sugar, or mixing in the syrup flavors and whipped cream, then just "forget about it," because that assumed health benefit is just not happening. Also, be sure to avoid the jelly donut with the coffee. That is a doctor-instructed "no-no."

For the lawyers in my family, let me phrase this carefully: As long as you do not suffer heart rhythm abnormalities or other caffeine-aggravated physical ailments (such as stomach ulcers or heartburn), consider adding a few cups of daily coffee brew. But at regular medical office visits, always review your habits with the medical provider to be sure that your coffee habit is a healthy habit. ☞

10 TIPS FOR TACKLING ACUTE BACK PAIN

As a spectator, I cringe a lot at football games. Not because my team is winning (Go Cowboys!) or losing, but because of the direct body impact these guys sustain during aggressive physical play. I also cringe a lot when I watch *America's Funniest Home Videos*. Those pitiful scenes when someone gets hurt tend to upset me more than make me laugh. My kids blame my "doctorness" (that is not a real word) and tell me I am an over-actor when I cover my face during the "funny" scenes. I just know those guys and gals hurt in the morning when they get out of bed (we won't even get into Tony Romo...). I wonder how many of them experience back pain.

New-onset low-back pain is what brings many patients into our clinic, and "acute" back-pain episodes are defined as six to 12 weeks of pain. Low-back pain is located between the mid- to low-back, and when pain radiates down one or both legs it is called sciatica.

For many readers this information seems repetitive, but here are some facts released by the American Academy of Family Practice that you will find interesting. (Some of it is new to me.)

1. First-time back-pain sufferers are usually between 20 and 40 years of age, and for many it is the first time to seek medical attention as an adult.
2. Approximately 31 percent of people with low-back pain do not fully recover within six months, but most will improve.

3. Pain returns in 25-62 percent of patients within one-two years. (What more can I say...)

4. Back pain could signal a significant underlying medical condition that should be ruled out by your medical provider. Tumors, kidney stones, vascular disease, bladder infections and bone marrow disorders are just a few of many diseases that present as sudden low-back pain.

5. Bed rest is not helpful for acute back pain. Over time, bed rest can promote joint stiffness and blood clots, in addition to muscle and bone mineral loss. Bed rest is also less effective at reducing pain and improving mobility than staying active.

6. For people with acute low-back pain, spinal manipulation, massage and chiropractic therapy do not improve outcomes of low-back pain; however, these methods may be beneficial for chronic back pain (yes, I said it and I will hear back from critics on this...).

7. While regular exercises may not help initially for acute low-back pain, certain forms of physical therapy may lessen the risk of its recurrence. (Look up the McKenzie method and its spine stabilization program achieved through physical therapy.)

8. Anti-inflammatory medicines are effective treatments for managing acute low-back pain. Over-the-counter ibuprofen and naproxen sodium are good examples of effective anti-inflammatories. Acetaminophen is not helpful for acute back pain.

9. Prescription muscle relaxants may be helpful for acute back pain. These medicines can comfort and relieve pain but will not shorten the duration of recovery.

10. In general, there is no need to order radiology imaging (x-rays, cat scans or MRI) for acute low-back pain unless other "red flag" signs or symptoms of more significant underlying problems are present. For example, sudden back pain in a 70-year-old lady with thin bones (osteoporosis) could indicate a spinal compression fracture

(bone collapse) and, at minimum, she would need an x-ray.

11. Heat works better than ice for acute low back pain. (BONUS—I'm giving you 11 facts... sorry, but I got carried away.) We have been conditioned to use ICE for early injury care, but in the case of the low spine, heat seems to work better. I should add that there is little evidence that supports the use of acupuncture, exercise, back support devices or traction to reduce acute back pain. But these are modalities that could be beneficial for chronic (ongoing) back pain beyond the three-month time marker.

Many times, staying at home, using heat and anti-inflammatories* and maintaining usual activities as tolerated is the best care for acute back pain. However, if pain worsens, begins to extend down the leg or is accompanied by fever, you should seek help through your medical provider. If you have a history of cancer, it is highly important you follow up to ensure there is no cancer recurrence in your bones. When in doubt, it does not hurt to seek medical advice.

*You should always discuss with your medical provider whether anti-inflammatories are safe in combination with your prescription medications or your ongoing medical problems.

> *Hug a hound!*
> The "pet effect" is real. Researchers found that people experienced lower blood pressures and stress while petting and talking to dogs.
> Journal of Behavioral Medicine Oct 1988

YOU MAY NOT BE ALLERGIC TO PENICILLIN

In the two decades since I was a resident, there have been no significant new antibiotics for patients in the clinic setting. Routine (and affordable) antibiotics for severe respiratory and intestinal and bladder/kidney infections have not significantly changed since I began private practice.

While we have managed to care well for our patients, we have limited choices of antibiotics. More and more (it seems), patients have developed specific antibiotic allergies, most particularly to penicillin. Recently a patient presented me with a dilemma. He needed an antibiotic for a kidney infection, but my treatment options were limited due to his multiple drug allergies. There were three classes of antibiotics that I could not use due to his specific drug reactions. I held my breath as I wrote a prescription for a non-standard antibiotic, praying it would achieve its healing purpose. Deep down I wondered, is he really allergic to all these antibiotics and what type of allergic reaction did he experience with each one?

A recent report in Asia Pacific Allergy journal (April 2013) found that approximately 10 percent of patients report penicillin allergies, yet only 10 percent have a proven penicillin reaction.

Many patients tell me they think—or were told—that they may have developed a rash from penicillin when they were children or that members of their family were allergic to penicillin. But it is common for children to develop skin eruptions with certain viruses. For example, many childhood rashes could easily be confused with a penicillin-allergy rash. Once the suspicious rash becomes associated with the antibiotic, we emblazon a person's medical chart with a permanent "red flag" penicillin-allergy "tattoo." This is done to ensure patient safety.

Anaphylactic shock from penicillin can be scary, and patients may come in to our medical facility with shortness of breath, severe rash and chest pain. In severe cases, the affected patient will stop breathing. Without immediate medical intervention, organ systems such as the brain, heart and kidneys lose blood flow, and death can occur. According to a Cleveland Clinic study, 500-1,000 deaths annually are attributable to penicillin allergies.

Luckily, severe penicillin reactions are uncommon. As it turns out, many patient-reported drug "allergies" are common antibiotic side effects such as diarrhea, nausea or stomach discomfort. However, it is critically important that your medical professional be certain that your drug allergy does not include a history of skin or respiratory symptoms, which are far more significant and potentially dangerous. If your reactions are mild, it will be up to you and your doctor to discern whether penicillin may be a future treatment option.

How do you know if you are truly allergic to penicillin? Skin testing is an option (under close physician observation), but a three-day oral challenge is the test more highly recommended (according to the Asia Pacific Allergy study). I would not recommend participation in penicillin-allergy testing if you might have had a severe allergic reaction such as severe rash, chest tightness, etc. However, if you have a questionable penicillin allergy, it may be worth a trip to your neighborhood allergist.

But why go to the trouble? If you were able to choose a low-cost penicillin-based drug instead of a highly complex alternative medication, you could potentially save money with less expensive penicillin-based antibiotics and reduce your risk for drug resistance. If you are repeatedly prescribed highly powerful (non-penicillin) antibiotics for minor infections, they may become less effective over time.

The bottom line: Discuss any penicillin allergies with your medical provider. Ask if you are a candidate for penicillin-allergy testing and review the risks and benefits of testing for a penicillin allergy and future use of penicillin-based medications. A 90 percent chance of NOT being allergic to penicillin makes for good odds (even outside of Las Vegas!). If you have had a severe reaction to penicillin, however, it is NOT worth playing Russian roulette. Leave it alone. However, a history of a possible minor penicillin drug reaction could make drug-allergy testing worth the potential wealth of future treatment options. ☛

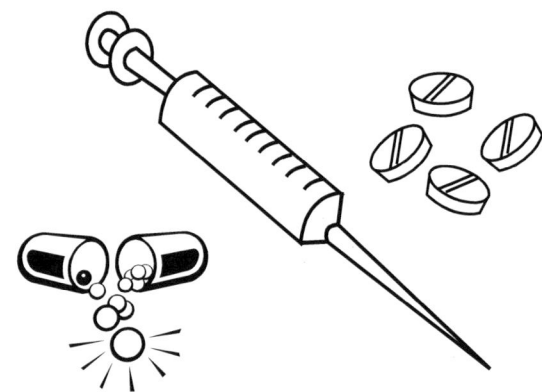

TIME FOR YOUR PHYSICAL!
BUT WHAT IF YOUR DOCTOR FINDS SOMETHING WRONG?

Trending...the annual physical. It is crunch time, and many patients have to get their routine exams scheduled by the end of the year. November and December are busy months here at the family practice clinic for routine medical exams, pap smears, mammograms, blood analyses and other tests.

I will go out on a limb and tell you that healthy patients generally expect "normal" results. But what if the clinical findings or tests are not normal?

A few weeks ago, I discovered an irregular heart rhythm in a 50-year-old otherwise-healthy gentleman. Understandably, he was surprised. "What do you mean my heart rate is abnormal? Was it abnormal last year?" I explained that his physical exam had changed from prior years. "Dr. Sadler, I come here yearly, have my physical exam, and you tell me it is normal." Yes, that is true. But, today (I gently explained), it is not normal, and we need to proceed with further heart testing. He was so taken aback, it was not until several days later that he called to set up his heart testing.

His reaction is not surprising. Several times a week we have to call and notify patients about their abnormal mammograms, pap smears or prostate studies (among many other abnormal test findings). To avoid the "shock" patients feel after we reveal unexpected abnormalities in routine tests, I have come up with softer interpretative terminology.

For example, "Your mammogram was not entirely normal. There was a small area or density that we need to more closely evaluate and ensure your mammogram is absolutely fine." This is gentler than saying, "Your mammogram is abnormal and we need to order more tests."

Abnormal pap smears are also difficult to report because patients expect these tests to be normal. They don't expect a phone call from their medical provider describing an abnormal pap smear and the necessity of biopsies to better determine the severity of their abnormal results. Patients may expect the annual physical to be a quick in and out event. But sometimes it is not.

The routine medical exam is purposeful. As a physician, I would love to tell everyone that their labs were "perfect"! However, be prepared to discuss any atypical findings with your medical provider. Yes, you will be surprised if you are called with abnormal results. But be prepared to act on those findings and be sure you follow up completely on subsequent recommended testing. ☛

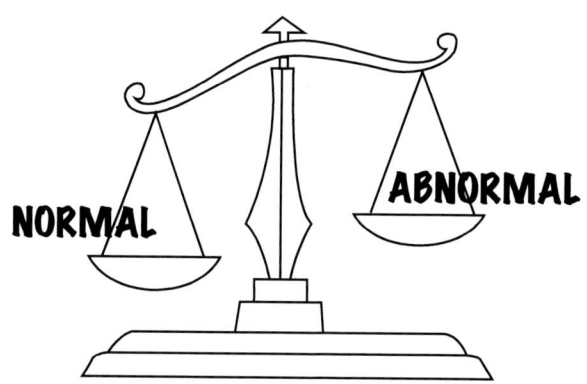

POOR TEXTING POSTURE IS A PAIN IN THE NECK

Is your teen complaining of periodic head and neck pain? Are YOU having more headaches and neck pain than in the past? You may want to evaluate your texting posture.

Seriously, look in the mirror while you conduct standard texting and take a "selfie." Then estimate the angle of the tilt of your head and neck. According to a study from Surgical Technology International (2014), poor posture associated with texting may add between 10-60 pounds of stress on the neck.

For example, without any tilt on the neck (0 degrees), resting pressure is simply the weight of the head (between 10-12 pounds). But for every 15 degrees of tilt there is an incremental increase in pounds of stress. With very poor posture, neck tension can reach up to 60 pounds. That is a full-sized monkey on your back!

Your neck is at its happiest in the C-curve. By angling forward to text, you reverse the natural C-curve, creating stress on the spine and promoting degenerative changes that will lead to early arthritis.

Of course, the spinal surgeons would love to see you once you start developing neurological issues related to severe neck arthritis and slipped cervical discs. This condition is called cervical radiculopathy. But why not avoid the pain and discomfort by texting healthier, starting now?

Sit up straight, tuck your stomach in tight, keep your shoulders back and place your phone at eye level. While it may seem awkward at first, this is the optimal position for texting. Good luck instructing your texting teen, but gentle reminders may be helpful over time.

If you or your teen have already developed "text neck," Dean Fishman, D.C., a chiropractor and the doctor who first coined this condition, offers exercises to combat the stress and strain of neck pain associated with texting. Pilates and yoga are also excellent ways to combat neck tension and improve posture awareness. ☛

> Did not get the childhood chicken pox rash? Most likely you still suffered the chicken pox virus. Up to 99% of adults 40 and older have had chicken pox in the past and many do not remember having the classic blistering rash. Do not take chances and go get the shingles vaccine. However, the vaccine's effectiveness wanes after five years and if you receive it before age 60, you should consider a booster. Discuss immunization options with your medical provider.
> www.vaccines.gov

HOLIDAY FEASTS MAY LEAD TO 'HOLIDAY HEART'

Ho-ho-NO! We all love the turkey, ham, gravy and holiday goodies that go along with this time of year. However, these food festivities may be responsible for the 14 percent increase in post-holiday hospitalizations for heart failure. Dr. Mahek Shah, a heart expert from Einstein Medical Center, coined the phrase "holiday heart" after a 10-year intensive review of hospital admission rates for heart failure on the days following Christmas.

He and his team at the medical center found that hospital admission rates for heart failure were 14 percent higher on Dec. 26-29 compared to routine daily admissions. His team found that daily admission rates for heart failure were higher after other celebratory events, too. Admissions were 11.4 percent higher July 5-8 and 11 percent higher on the four days after Super Bowl Sunday.

According to the Centers for Disease Control and Prevention (CDC), about 5.1 million people in the U.S. suffer from heart failure and heart failure is responsible for one in nine deaths. Approximately 50 percent of people diagnosed with heart failure will die within five years of initial diagnosis.

Dr. Shah suspects that holiday heart is likely due to celebratory habits that include overindulging in fatty and salt-laden foods. In addition, some heart-failure patients may be away from home and might delay seeking medical care in order to avoid interfering with family holiday plans.

My best medical advice? Push away from the table before you get full, put away the salt shaker, and do your best to avoid salty and fatty foods. I understand this is very difficult to do and that food has always been associated with celebratory events. But be smart and go for a heart-healthy diet. ☛

> The DASH Diet for Dummies, written by my sister, cardiologist Sarah Samaan, M.D., is an excellent reference for all of us and would be a great holiday gift for anyone suffering from heart failure.

MULTITASKING IS BAD FOR THE BRAIN (AND MY DAUGHTER'S IPHONE)

My daughter just broke her third iPhone 6. She was baking, talking, intermittently texting and cleaning at the same time. Of course, it was not her fault she placed the heavy mixer on top of her phone (I am being facetious). Unfortunately the cast-iron mixer not only destroyed her phone case and cracked the lens, but it rendered the home button completely inoperable.

I have to take some credit for this teen tragedy. Her multitasking tendency is probably a result of years of observing and perfecting my own bad habit. My husband has warned my daughter and me that our multitasking creates inefficiencies. He is right, and now she is paying for it (literally).

My daughter and I are not alone in our misgivings. There are many high-level multitaskers out there, so take heed. Media technology continues to advance, creating more multitaskers who will experience more and more challenges to their cognitive control. Proceeding of the National Academy of Sciences (August 2014) confirms that the brain performance of high-level multitaskers suffered when put to tasks similar to low-level multitaskers. It seems they are more susceptible to distractions and therefore perform less well at similar tasks when compared to people who take on one task at a time.

Lessons learned (and still learning). Did I mention that she has gone through 22 phones in her lifetime, and employees at the phone center know her on a first-name basis? I hope that iPhone is insured. And, what is she doing with an iPhone 6 when I have a 5? I could tell some stories, but I do not want to put my parenting skills under any more scrutiny! ☛

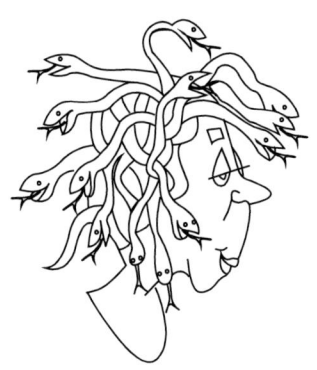

WANT THE NEW YEAR TO BEGIN HEALTHIER? THINK YOGURT!

I have had the same breakfast for the last 30 years. No kidding. Ever since college, I have enjoyed my cup of coffee yogurt in the morning. Heck, sometimes I even throw on some whipped cream (people add cream to their coffee, right?).

My children find this ritual strange, my husband just knows I am quirky, and most of my friends don't know about my coffee yogurt obsession.

Today, I can be proud of my healthy habit (minus the whipped cream) and be confident that continuing my daily yogurt consumption will be beneficial in the long run. According to a recent study, higher intake of yogurt was associated with a lower risk of type 2 diabetes. In addition, the study found that there was a dose-response relationship with yogurt. With more servings of daily yogurt, the risk of diabetes dropped even more.

One daily serving (defined as only 2 tablespoons, or 28 grams) was linked to an 18 percent reduction in the risk of type 2 diabetes. For comparison, there are approximately 170 grams in a (fruit-on-the-bottom) Dannon yogurt single-serve container. Therefore this study from BioMed Central Medicine (December 2014) suggests a healthy incremental benefit from eating yogurt every day.

The study, conducted by a team out of the Harvard School of Public Health, reviewed data from three larger studies that had collected information on dairy food intake from more than 195,000 health professionals. Over several decades' time, approximately 15,000 participants developed type 2 diabetes. That is a significant number of diabetics.

According to the Centers for Disease Control and Prevention (CDC), approximately 9.3 percent of Americans have diabetes (about 29 million people). Any positive impact on these numbers could significantly impact quality of life and health care costs. The average annual cost of health care for people with diabetes (2009) was $11,700 (CDC.gov). For diabetics with kidney complications, the average cost was closer to $20,000.

Most Americans are searching for ways to cut health care costs. However, if you are not a yogurt fan, this blog may seem less important to you. Unfortunately, researchers found no association with other dairy foods and reductions of type 2 diabetes risks. In other words, ice cream is not on the healthy list. For me, this investigation reinforces that having coffee yogurt for breakfast is my daily dose of healthy indulgence. I hope you find yours. ☛

EGG-CITING NEWS FOR PEOPLE WHO LOVE EGGS

I love eggs. I especially love the yolk. Do not expect me to share this perfectly round, golden nugget with anyone, because it is highly palatable. As far as the egg white, I usually give that to my kids or the dogs. My daughter insists the egg whites are healthier. Subsequently, she and I share our eggs. She eats the whites because they are "healthier" and I enjoy the delicious yolks. When it comes to eggs, my daughter and I are highly efficient eaters. This latest news, however, may change my daughter's mind about her yolk-aversion.

Much to everyone's surprise, traditional dietary guidelines centered on decreasing dietary cholesterol are being debunked. Egg yolks are no longer considered a "nutrient of concern." Other foods high in cholesterol such as shrimp and lobster are also being released from the bad-for-you food list, although foods high in fats such as butter, heavy cream and fatty foods remain under dietary restriction.

In a recent study, consumption of one egg daily did not increase the risk of heart disease. Even more promising, higher egg consumption was associated with a 25 percent reduction of stroke in one subset of study participants. In addition, previous studies found that increasing dietary cholesterol intake had very little impact in approximately 70 percent of people. In many people, high blood cholesterol levels are hereditary and may not be significantly affected by cholesterol-lowering diets. However, there are other diets and lifestyle changes that can help to improve health.

Guidelines from 2010 recommended cholesterol consumption of less than 300 mg per day. The average egg contains approximately 200 mg of cholesterol. Most omelets contain two-three eggs, which exceeds prior nutritional cholesterol recommendations. This doctor is not providing full medical clearance (yet) to binge on daily omelets made with two-three eggs, but that may change if studies continue to support the egg's healthy nutritional status. Be a responsible egg eater. Anything fried cannot be good for you!

To my family: You know all those cartons of egg whites we have in the refrigerator? Can we finally ditch them and have regular whole-egg omelets? They taste much better and (in limited quantities) are just fine for healthy eating!

BREAKING HEALTHY

My daughter is gluten-free, my husband is low-carb, and my son and I are hungry. At my house, we have jars of chia seeds, walnuts, almonds, pumpkin seeds and unidentifiable healthy-appearing food items. In addition, the fridge is full of soy, almond and cashew milk (who knew?). All the cheese and yogurt is fat-free.

I suppose I should not complain. My LDL (bad cholesterol) dropped about 25 points in the past year and my HDL (good cholesterol) jumped about 30 points, making an already excellent cholesterol panel even more incredible (I boast). I was amazed. Why? How? Despite indulging myself with a stash of coveted Cheetos and decadent dark-chocolate treats, I had managed to improve my cholesterol profile.

I have been skeptical about healthy dietary changes and their link to improved blood cholesterol levels. In clinical practice, modest improvements generally are seen with significant weight loss. Otherwise, most diets have not proven as successful as my personal experience at home. Are my patients telling the truth about their "healthier" diets, or are my family's healthier lifestyle choices a better way to improve cholesterol numbers?

Studies show that eating 30 grams of walnuts a day can improve HDL levels, and eating nuts up to four times weekly may decrease the risk of heart attack by as much as 40 percent.

Nuts can be safely introduced early in life. According to a well-publicized New England Journal of Medicine editorial (February 2015), approximately 2 percent of children have peanut allergies, but the article reaffirms prior evidence that introducing peanut-based products within the first year of life to healthy children may decrease peanut allergies up to 80 percent.

However, before an infant sticks fingers into the peanut butter jar, be certain your medical provider approves. Some children are especially prone to nut-based food allergies and are not candidates for nut-based proteins.

The American Heart Association recommends four servings of unsalted nuts a week. One serving of raw nuts, defined as 1-1/2 ounces, is equivalent to approximately 30 almonds, 21 walnut halves, 25 cashews, 60 pistachios or two tablespoons of nut butter.

At 160 to 190 calories per ounce, the caloric costs can be high. While nuts have high calorie concentrations, they are likely to lower body weight and fat mass in overweight people while decreasing risks for diabetes (British Journal of Nutrition, 2006). In addition, this research suggests that adding nuts to our diet produces longer-lasting weight loss and a "greater magnitude" of successful weight loss compared with alternative low-fat diets.

Obvious doctor advice: Avoid overindulging on the delicious, aromatic, candied nuts like those hard-to-resist (and my favorite) cinnamon almonds sold at the great State Fair of Texas.

Meanwhile, my family continues to rely on its low-carb, low-gluten, high nut-based diet. Flexing my diet to fit in with the family is not new to me. (This is not my first rodeo.) I fondly recall early experiences on the family farm in Cat Spring, Texas. My well-meaning father sent my pet steer, Lone Ranger, to the meatpacking plant and then straight to our freezer. In rebellion over this terrible tragedy, my three sisters and I, along with our mother, stopped eating red meat and became vegetarians. Our diets relied heavily on nuts and fish.

Eventually, most of us girls went back to our carnivorous food habits, but to this day my mother remains a vegetarian cattle rancher.

At home, my husband cooks, so I have limited food choices due to his (and my daughter's) healthy dietary choices. I'm somewhat of a rebel and insist on adding whipped cream to my fat-free yogurt. And today, as I do frequently now, I will pick up my son from school, glance over at him and casually ask, "How about a Whataburger for the drive home?" ☞

LOW FAT   *Low Carb*   **GLUTEN FREE**

High Protein   **SUGAR FREE**

HOW COLD? EQUESTRIAN PANNICULITIS COLD!

Seen by a doctor and unsuccessfully treated, the woman was understandably frustrated when she came to us for a second opinion. I had no idea what had caused her unusual blotchy, blue and cold rash. Its odd distribution was limited to her horse-rider's saddle-seat, which made this rash exceptionally puzzling. It was not a bruise or an allergic reaction. It was "prickly" but not itching. What in the world was going on here?

My usual medical go-to websites and dermatology books were useless. I shamefully admit that I succumbed to a Google search for help. No answers.

Not one to waste time, I rushed to the phone and called Dr. Kendra Rorrie because she is brilliant. According to my dermatology friend, the history and rash were diagnostic of equestrian cold panniculitis. I never heard of it. She explained that the unusual condition is one that many dermatologists have studied but most never see in clinical practice (or at least here in our usually warmer Texas winters).

Equestrian cold panniculitis is a result of prolonged cold exposure while seated in the saddle. Wet and cold weather (like what we are currently experiencing) can promote decreased blood flow and inflammation in the superficial fatty tissue of the thigh, buttocks and lower abdomen. In one study, four patients were young, healthy women equestrians who rode at least two hours daily. Their uninsulated, tight-fitting riding pants slowed blood flow through covered areas of the skin, causing small, red, itchy lesions on the upper and outer portions of both thighs. In some study patients, the rash became more severe and progressed to tender bumps and raised painful plaques. Fortunately, my patient's condition was far less severe.

Cold panniculitis is not limited to horse riders. It has also been reported in cyclists, golf-cart riders and milk-delivery men (they do exist in Finland!). In infants, the rash can be found on cheeks and forehead—so keep those babies covered up against the cold!

My patient is a dedicated equestrian and regularly exercises seven horses daily. We compromised and I cleared her to return to riding but only with "prescribed" breathable-cotton long johns under her riding pants. Today, I called to check on her. Unfortunately, she is not keeping up her end of the bargain, but that is OK. As a former equestrian, I understand how difficult it can be to put anything under those tight riding pants! At least she now understands her medical condition and knows how to best manage her discomfort if her panniculitis worsens over the next few cold, wintery days.

> Of the top 125 school ranked in U.S. News and World Report, 48% of them have tanning beds on or near campus.
>
> Journal of the American Medical Association (JAMA) Dermatology October 2015.

IS THERE A DOCTOR ON THE PLANE?
(OR, MEDICAL CONDITIONS THAT DON'T FLY WELL)

"Is there a doctor on the plane? We have a medical emergency!"

I was sleeping hard on the soft pillow put in front of me. Fortunately, since residency training an emergency call in the middle of a deep sleep has always turned on the adrenaline release and enabled me to awaken quickly.

The 39-year-old gentleman had fainted but was conscious by the time I reached his seat. Nearby passengers selflessly gave up their seats, and I was able to lay my sickened patient flat as the flight attendant brought the on-flight medical bag.

Blood pressure was low, pulse was slightly high, color was pale, but he improved over the next several minutes. This healthy father of seven had no significant medical history other than having recently donated blood and a mild cold.

By the time the plane was ready for landing, he was still unable to sit up comfortably, and it became obvious he would need immediate further medical attention. Once on the ground in Denver, the airport promptly delivered its "A-team" paramedics, and he was transported to a medical facility for observation and care.

Diagnosis? Most likely my in-flight patient had suffered vasovagal syncope as a result of dehydration from a recent-onset viral illness. The blood transfusion from two weeks earlier was only a "red herring," or what we medical people call interesting but non-relevant history (healthy people screened for blood transfusions generally will not have symptoms related to donating blood). His illness and lack of fluids may have caused a drop in blood pressure, which can cause nausea and dizziness and, in severe cases, lead to loss of consciousness. It is one of the more common in-flight emergencies, according to the Centers for Disease Control and Prevention (CDC).

Four other common in-flight medical emergencies (in order of frequency) include gastrointestinal, respiratory, cardiology and neurologic events. The CDC suggests that some people may experience worsening of uncontrolled lung disease (such as asthma or COPD), sickle cell disease and untreated anemia, and should exercise caution before flying. People with uncontrolled blood pressure, a recent stroke or recent surgery should consult with their medical provider before boarding a plane.

About one in 10,000 to 40,000 passengers suffer a medical incident and one in 150,000 requires the use of in-flight medicine or medical equipment. The CDC estimates annual deaths aboard commercial aircraft to be 0.3 per 1 million passengers. About one-third of these are due to heart conditions.

Because the paramedics were busy assisting the man, I was unable to provide him with my own contact information before he was taken from the airplane. I plan to call the airline to follow up on his condition. As a father of seven, my patient certainly needs to get back on his feet quickly, although I am sure he needs an excuse for some well-deserved rest.

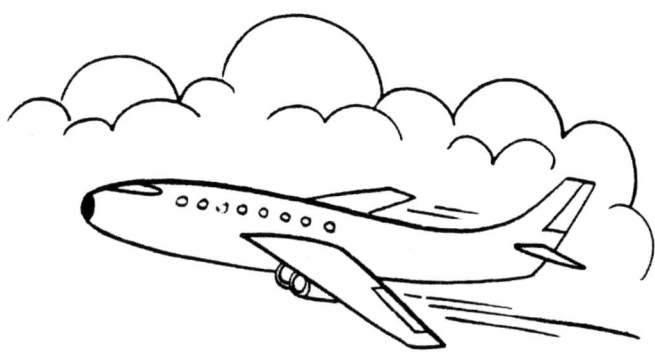

A CLUTTERED ROOM AND A CLUTTERED MIND

Their rooms are untidy and their clothes are on the floor. This is not the way to run a household. Both kids are not attending to their chores and I am frustrated. During the summer (it is bliss), my kids take care of dishes, laundry, floors and dog poop. I give them a little break during school time. They are only required to maintain good grades, keep their rooms clean and pick up dog poop.

I am obsessed at maintaining an orderly house (that is not so orderly at all). My kids think I have an obsessive-compulsive problem, but there is method to my madness because a strong correlation exists between cleanliness and academic performance. A 2008 study from the Association of Higher Education polled 1,481 students, and 88 percent reported a lack of cleanliness as a significant academic distraction. Cleanliness ranked fourth among the most important environmental factors to impact a student's personal learning.

"Clutter in space is like cluttering your mind," according to psychologist Brandi Sinclair, LPC, with Heritage Counseling and Consulting in Dallas. Brandi recognizes that having a disorganized room creates a feeling of inefficiency. "Life is managing you, and you are not managing your life," she says.

Clean up your work space, too. Living without environmental chaos applies to both adults and children. ☛

WHAT DO BROKEN MIRRORS AND HOT FLASHES HAVE IN COMMON? 7 HOT FLASH FACTS

Seven years: The average time hot flashes continue past the final menstrual cycle. For many unfortunate women, reaching menopause may be like breaking a mirror and winding up with seven years of bad luck.

However, like an extra-small pair of Spanx, this seven-year hot flash glove is not one-size-fits all. Some lucky women float coolly through the menopause maze, getting nowhere close to the fire.

JAMA Internal Medicine (February 2015) has published a large study that finds that frequent post-menopausal symptoms including hot flashes and night sweats (VMS: vasomotor symptoms) lasted an average of more than seven years. Importantly, the large-scale study revealed that VMS significantly affected the quality of life for most women and that numbers of "broken mirror" years varied between groups of women.

Seven fascinating hot-flash facts released in this study include:

1. About 80 percent of women experience VMS during the menopausal transitional years.
2. The median VMS duration for women across all ethnicities was 7.4 years.
3. Women who experienced VMS symptoms early on in their perimenopausal years were more likely to suffer the longest total duration of VMS, with a median time frame of more than 11.8 years and continued VMS after the final menstrual period of 9.4 years.

4. Good news for those beyond periods at the onset of VMS: These lucky women had the shortest duration of symptoms, with only 3.4 years of VMS after their final menstrual period.

5. African-American women experienced the longest duration of hot flashes, lasting up to a median of 10.1 years.

6. Japanese and Chinese women had the shortest duration of hot flashes (4.8 and 5.4 median years, respectively).

7. Longer duration of VMS was found more often in women who were a younger age at menopause, had lower educational status or had greater "perceived stress." In addition, higher depression and anxiety levels were linked to longer duration of VMS.

So where is the answer to "What can I do to treat my hot flashes?" I wish I could tell you I had the key to that door. Hormone replacement therapy may reduce VMS symptoms but is not considered safe for all women, including those with a history of stroke or breast cancer (for example). For my patients, the general rule for hormone replacement therapy is "the lowest dose for the shortest period of time necessary to treat symptoms." Long-term hormone therapy may put some women at risk for breast cancer, varicose veins, blood clots and more.

There are, however, other (less effective) options to treat VMS. Some manufactured low-dose antidepressants have been approved and marketed to women suffering moderate to severe hot flashes. For example, at a 57-59 percent reduction of VMS, Brisdelle is marginally favorable to a placebo, which comes in at a close second at 40-48 percent effectiveness.

Bottom line: Vasomotor symptoms related to hot flashes unfavorably impact quality of life. It is time to find long-lasting, safe relief that can be better tolerated than 7.4 years of heat. ☛

BATS BITE IN THE SPRING (NOT JUST HALLOWEEN)

Opening the umbrella on an outdoor table seems like a safe and mindless mission. But it can be more complicated if you bother the sleeping bat inside the oversized umbrella. My patient described the unpleasant (and disturbing) experience: the blood running down her finger, her protective, quick-thinking husband managed to trap the sun-stunned bat until Garland Animal Control arrived. Kudos to all!

A patient with a bat bite is an unexpected physical complaint for a Saturday morning clinic. However, family practice days can be (with a nod to Forrest Gump) like a box of chocolates. You never know what you are going to get when you open the exam-room door. My obvious concern was for rabies transmission in this otherwise healthy young woman. There was no time to waste; it was time to consult the Centers for Disease Control (CDC) for treatment strategy. Thank you, Internet (and my infectious-disease specialist friend, Dr. Claire Brenner with Baylor Garland)!

The last time I gave rabies shots was more than 10 years ago. Obtaining necessary human immune globulin and rabies vaccine quickly is vitally important, and the window of treatment is narrow. Rabies is 100 percent fatal without early intervention. Understandably, the complexity of treatment strategy can be overwhelming for both patients and clinicians.

The CDC claims there are only one or two human rabies cases annually. Between 1967 and 2006, there were 19 cases of human rabies, of which 17 were associated with bats. Thankfully, many thousands of people bitten by rabid animals are successfully treated through vaccination. In most cases of rabies death, people who died did not know they had been bitten. According to the CDC, rabies in humans is 100 percent preventable through prompt "appropriate medical care."

The CDC described early rabies symptoms as being similar to those of the flu virus. Initially presenting symptoms include general weakness, malaise, fever and headache. Progression of the disease results in anxiety, confusion, irritability, abnormal behavior and hallucinations. By this time, the disease has progressed beyond reversible stages and death is imminent.

Thankfully, our bat was rapidly transported to Austin and its brain tissue was immediately evaluated for the presence of rabies virus antigens. Within 48 hours we had our results: negative for rabies. What an efficient system our state and local government have for disease management! ☞

> According to the American Academy of Dermatology, people who first use tanning beds before age 35 are 75% more likely to develop skin melanoma.
>
> Cancer Epidemiology, Biomarkers & Prevention
> May 2010

8 SIGNS THAT YOUR HEALTHY EATING IS MAKING YOU SICK

You cannot eat a bite of your birthday cake? Obsessed with eating gluten-free or low-carbohydrate foods? Do your all-consuming (pardon the pun) efforts to eat chemical-free meats, fats and artificial additives adversely affect your social life and hinder your ability to think beyond your next meal?

If not, then don't worry. However, if nutritional issues unnaturally intrude on your daily activities and social life, you could be orthorexic.

It has been called a "fixation on righteous eating" or an unnatural obsession with maintaining a healthy diet. Orthorexia, according to the National Eating Disorders Association (NEDA), is not recognized yet as a formal clinical diagnosis, although it is seen in clinical practice. Orthorexia is when a person's self-esteem depends on the adherence to a restrictive healthy diet. As opposed to anorexia nervosa, orthorexics obsess with healthy eating and not with losing weight, being thin or having a certain body image. According to NEDA, an orthorexic's healthy food obsessions can impair the ability to engage in usual activities and relationships.

Being too strict in dietary selections may be harmful. Orthorexics may have nutritionally defective diets that lack specific vitamins and minerals. Nutritional support by a professional dietitian generally is recommended. Are you at risk for orthorexia? NEDA offers eight questions to help you find out. The more "yes" answers, the more likely you could be an orthorexic.

1. Do you wish that occasionally you could just eat and not worry about food quality?
2. Do you ever wish you could spend less time on food and more time living and loving?
3. Does it seem beyond your ability to eat a meal prepared with love by someone else and not try to control what is served?
4. Are you constantly looking for ways foods are unhealthy for you?
5. Do love, joy, play and creativity take a back seat to following the perfect diet?
6. Do you feel guilt or self-loathing when you stray from your diet?
7. Do you feel in control when you stick to the "correct" diet?
8. Have you put yourself on a nutritional pedestal and wonder how others can possibly eat the foods they eat?

Professional medical attention generally is recommended, and many skilled counselors and nutritionists can help deal with orthorexia and its undesirable physical and psychosocial consequences. Admitting there is a problem, learning to accept dietary flexibility and dealing with any food-related emotional issues will help in recovery.

Self-esteem does not come by imposing highly selective healthy eating into one's lifestyle. Instead it comes from being a happy, self-confident person who seeks to incorporate more healthy lifestyles. After all, what is a birthday without a high-carbohydrate, gluten-full birthday cake and ice cream? ☞

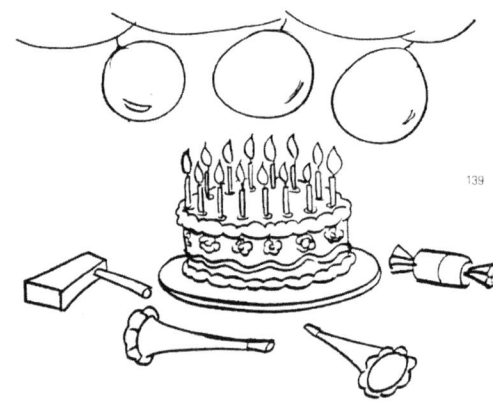

SOME FATS ARE NOT ALL THAT BAD AND SOME ARE THE BEE'S KNEES!

My friends scoff at my love of drinking half-and-half in coffee and lattes. To me, that added fat is the "bee's knees." So, let us settle two questions in this short (and written-late-at-night blog).

1. Is half-and-half really bad for me?
2. Do bees really have knees?

As a medical doctor, I have to think professionally and answer question number one first. An article in the American Journal of Clinical Nutrition (April 2015) found that many fat-rich proteins such as eggs, whole milk, full-fat cheese and nuts do not have a significant impact on weight gain. These fat-rich foods, generally avoided in low-fat diets, are less important to pass up for successful weight loss. Instead, adults should be more concerned about calories consumed in carbohydrate-laden foods such as breads, crackers, potatoes, sugary soda or fruit drinks.

According to the article, both the quantity and quality of carbohydrates seem to be most important to weight management. Labeled the glycemic load, this measurement can more easily compare and contrast carbohydrates and better prepare us for healthy choices to reduce our muffin tops (or maintain our shapely figures). MedlinePlus compares single servings of white-flour bagels with a glycemic load of 25 units to quinoa (pronounced keen-wah), with a glycemic index of 13, and chickpeas, with a glycemic index of 3. The lower the glycemic index the better, which makes this glycemic index approach more dietary specific and scientifically sophisticated when compared to simple caloric counts.

Perhaps we should not be so strict in reducing our kids' whole milk to 1 percent (who likes that watery substitute anyway?). Perhaps we should be more careful about the other foods they eat and let them have a little bit more peanut butter and more boiled eggs (yolks included).

Now, to answer question two: It is very difficult to find legitimate scientific articles about bees and their knees, but I think I have an answer. Bees do not actually have knees but they do have a femur and a tibia, which is what we humans call our thigh and shin bones (respectively). Without a hinged joint and knee-cap (patella), it would be very difficult to attest that bees have knees. The phrase, however, is cute and catchy, so I feel no need to remove the idiom from my vocabulary.

> *There are more skin cancer cases due to indoor tanning than lung cancer cases due to smoking.*
> *JAMA Dermatology January 2014*

10 LIFE-SAVING FACTS YOU NEED TO KNOW ABOUT LIGHTNING

Alone in the house and sleeping in after a late night of studying, she did not hear lightning strike the gas line. But Sam was abruptly awakened by an anxious dog. My poodle, Jett, had sensed something was not right. Unable to rest with the weight of a large standard poodle on her chest, my daughter forced herself out of a restful sleep and followed Jett down the stairs.

But Jett was not wanting her morning feed. She was restless, whiny and "really acting strange." Then Sam heard the sound: a crackle.

Moving closer to the fireplace, she heard gas coming from the fireplace. She attempted to close the gas line to the fireplace with the metal key. Strangely, the switch was already in the off position. Something was not right. Then Sam placed her hand on the wall and heat from a fire behind the wall singed her hand. Again, the sound: a second crackle, like the sound of fire. Quick to act, she dialed 911 and ran to get my neighbor. Together, they quickly evacuated the dogs from the house. The punctured gas line continued to leak dangerous fumes into our home. Then the Garland Fire Department arrived to save the day. My daughter tells me that their heroic call-to-response time was only three minutes. Thank you!

Lightning ignites 22,600 fires a year in the U.S., according to the National Fire Protection Agency. Some 4,290 of those fires involve homes. Between 2004 and 2008, only 18 percent of fires caused by lightning strikes occurred in homes, but these fires accounted for 88 percent of lightning-related deaths. Annually, lightning-related fires account for 53 injuries and 12 deaths (which includes at least nine or more of our rescue firefighters who die annually).

About 28 people die annually from direct lightning strikes. Deaths generally occur in an open area where there is no shelter. The National Weather Service has recommendations for lightning safety that should come in handy over the next several days when more thunderstorms are expected to hit our area. Here are a few:

1. When you hear thunder, immediately move to safe shelter: an enclosed building or a metal-topped vehicle with windows all the way up.
2. Stay in the shelter for at least 30 minutes after you hear the last sound of thunder.
3. Stay off corded phones, computers or electrical equipment that put you in direct contact with electricity.
4. Avoid plumbing, including sinks, baths and faucets.
5. Stay away from windows and doors and stay off the porch.
6. Do not lie on concrete floors and do not lean against concrete walls.
7. If you are outside, immediately get off elevated areas and never lie flat on the ground.
8. Do not seek shelter under an isolated tree and do not use a cliff or rocky overhand for shelter.
9. Immediately get out of and away from pools, ponds, lakes and other bodies of water.
10. Stay away from objects that could conduct electricity, such as barbed wire fences or power lines.

Again, I want to thank the Garland Fire Department's rapid response team (C shift: Stations 6, 7, 10 and 11). Your quick actions saved our home. To my dog, Jett, thank you, sweet friend, and praise the Lord for giving you insight into danger so that you were able to save the life of my precious daughter. ☛

ARE YOU ITCHING TO GET OUT IN THE SUN, OR DOES THE SUN MAKE YOU ITCH?

After weeks of wet weather, we are finally getting a breath of fresh, and rather warm, air. The Texas sun has made a return. Bring out your sunglasses and get outside for your therapeutic vitamin D and seasonal light therapy—it is sure to lift your mood!

But our Texas UV rays may be harmful, so strike a good balance. Too much sun exposure may lead to sunburns, heat-related dehydration and funny looking rashes.

Yes, rashes.

This past Sunday, people took to the sunny outdoors and many forgot their sunscreen and clothing cover-ups. Unfortunately, some are suffering for it. How do I know? This week many patients came into the clinic with complaints of itchy red bumps and blisters. Many of these outbreaks were in sun-exposed areas such as the arms and chest. Certainly the pain and swelling can be uncomfortable. These particular cases were consistent with hypersensitivity to the sun, a condition consistent with photodermatitis.

This skin irritation is a result of an altered immune system response to the sun's UV rays. This condition often runs in families but may occur due to environmental elements such as exposure to perfumes (especially those with lavender) and medications. Diuretic and antibiotic prescriptions such as those containing sulfa compounds (i.e., hydrochlorothiazide and Bactrim) could promote skin sensitivity with UV exposure.

Some herbs or edible plants can increase the risk for photodermatitis. Examples include celery, parsnip, carrots and hogweed (who eats that?). For a complete list, see UMM.edu.

You can prevent photodermatitis by applying PABA-free sunscreens with a sun protection factor (SPF) of 30. Higher SPF factors may not provide any more benefit (but that is a story for another day). Cover up with long-sleeved shirts, pants and a hat whenever possible. Some of the more recent clothing catalogs demonstrate fashionable long-sleeve bathing tops. Sometimes controlled clinical phototherapy to desensitize patients from the sun can help prevent future outbreaks.

For extremely irritated skin, cool, wet washcloths may provide temporary relief. Prescription medications such as oral steroids or azathioprine may be used if the symptoms warrant medical intervention.

Some occasions may warrant supplements such as vitamins C or D in cases of nutritional deficiencies. Occasionally, homeopathic herbal remedies such as rhodiola extract or astragalus extract may relieve symptoms. However, these herbs may interfere with prescription medications, and you should consult with your physician prior to using them.

Complications include risk for premature aging of the skin and an increased chance of developing dark patches from the use of a steroid cream or from chronic itching. Some people may be at higher risk for skin cancer. For most people, however, there is fun in the sun and nothing to worry about other than sunburns.

DO YOU ATTRACT OR REPEL MOSQUITOES? 7 HELPFUL MOSQUITO FACTS

Mosquitoes seem to avoid her. She is worried. A circulating "old wives' tale" suggests that mosquitoes avoid people with cancer and now her daughter is concerned. My initial reaction was to reassure the family and tell them not to lose sleep over silly nonsense. But doing some research gave me the curiosity bug (no pun intended).

According to CDC.gov, almost 40,000 U.S. residents have documented West Nile viral disease since 1999. Mosquito-borne West Nile virus is responsible for 17,000 serious illnesses and more than 1,600 deaths.

Thus the importance of this medical search: Do mosquitoes have selective sensors? Would they avoid some people and be more likely to bite others? I was a little taken aback by my findings:

1. Hereditary factors play a role in mosquito bite susceptibility. Studies found inherited factors, including natural body odor, may act as a natural repellent. Scientists found that mosquitoes avoided some individuals but were drawn to others. I agree that a structural nose would look funny on a mosquito. Actually, its sensory organ is housed in its well-hidden olfactory system.

2. Mosquitoes are drawn to people with blood type O almost twice as much as people with type A. People with type B fall somewhere in the middle. I could not, however, find affirmation of these studies by the Centers for Disease Control and Prevention (CDC).

3. Using DEET (N, N-Diethyl-meta-toluamide) can repel mosquitoes. However, one study found that more than half of *Aedes aegypti* mosquitoes (most common in North America) developed resistance to DEET's deterrent properties. Other DEET-exposed species have shown up to a 10 percent DEET resistance. DEET can be an effective mosquito repellent, but clearly other options should be considered, including wearing loose, long-sleeve clothing, using mosquito nets or applying less-potent repellents.

4. Plant-based oil of lemon eucalyptus is another repellent approved by the CDC and the Environmental Protection Agency. I am sure this smells better than DEET. It may be my "go to" repellent spray. Essential oils such as "pure oil of lemon eucalyptus" are not individually approved, although the inclusion of oil of lemon eucalyptus with other ingredients (in Repel and Off, for example) may increase its efficacy.

5. Mosquitoes carrying West Nile virus tend to bite late in the day. Cover up and use protective mosquito repellent if you plan to be outdoors between dusk and dawn.

6. Mosquitoes are attracted to pregnant women and overweight people because of their increased emissions of carbon dioxide (CO_2). They are less likely to bite skinny people and children.

7. Mosquitoes love sweaty people. Lactic acid, secreted during high levels of physical activity, may naturally repel the opposite sex but is a natural mosquito attractant. If you are outside in the heat, be sure to reapply your insect repellent periodically, as body sweat will dilute its potent properties.

Mosquitoes love moist weather, and much-needed rain has recently come to Texas in great abundance. Along with this unanticipated monsoon season, I anticipate a highly active mosquito summer. We are already seeing several patients with multiple stings, so adequately prepare before heading out into our city—or, should I say, the "Dallas rainforest."

As far as my patient's question, there is some anecdotal information on the Internet that suggests certain cancer chemotherapy drugs (probably drugs that increase CO_2 excretion) could repel mosquitos. But there is no available literature to suggest mosquitoes prefer cancer patients over anyone else. Either way, I hope this blog has addressed my patient's concerns and that she finds this information reassuring. ☛

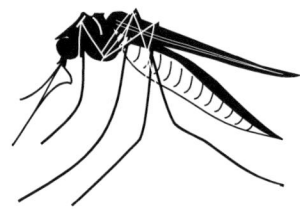

7 SOUR TRUTHS ABOUT SWEETENED BEVERAGES

In my clinic, kids look forward to their "Sadler snacks" as a special award for great behavior. The delicious fruity drinks and gummy snacks are well loved by my little patients. I keep plenty of bottled water for a more healthy option, but the juice usually wins out. While my legendary Sadler snacks bring plenty of smiles, I shamefully admit they pack on plenty of unnecessary, sugary calories.

Recently Channel 4 contacted me for an interview about a study on sugary drinks. Intrigued by the research, I wanted to go back after my brief television interview and learn more. I could not help but feel a twinge of guilt because of my sweet-snack distributions. Nonetheless, I have come up with seven interesting—yet "bitter"—facts about sweetened beverages that summarize why this information matters to you:

1. Worldwide, sugary drinks may be responsible for up to 184,000 deaths annually, including 25,000 deaths in the United States. Latin America had the most deaths from sugary drinks. Mexico, for example experiences an estimated 24,000 deaths annually as a result of these sweet treats. Tufts University's research model, published in the journal Circulation (June 2015), estimates that around the world, sugared drinks lead to 133,000 deaths from diabetes, 45,000 deaths from heart disease and 6,450 deaths from cancer.

2. In the U.S., two out of three adults and one out of three children are obese or overweight.

3. People who regularly consume one-two cans of sweetened drinks daily have a 26 percent increase in the risk of developing type 2 diabetes.

4. Over 20 years, consuming just one sugary beverage daily may increase the risk of heart attack by up to 20 percent.

5. The National Cancer Institute links obesity to increased risk for multiple cancer types, including esophageal, pancreatic, colorectal, uterine, breast (post-menopausal), thyroid, kidney and gallbladder.

6. A 12-ounce cola contains approximately 10 teaspoons of sugar. The average American consumes 22 teaspoons of sugar daily. A Harvard Letter review summarized studies linking sugary drinks to obesity. Children who consumed an average of one 12-ounce soda daily developed a 60 percent increased risk for obesity within an 18-month period.

7. According to Tufts University, Mexico had the highest population of deaths contributed to overconsumption of sugary drinks: 30 percent in people under age 45. On the other hand, deaths in Japan from sugar drinks were minimal because the Japanese are more accustomed to drinking unsweetened teas.

The Tufts University researchers' conclusions are based on sugary drink consumption trends, death rates and sugar availability.

Perhaps we should all put down the colas. Considering artificially sweetened beverages? Think again. Go back to my blog about diet drinks (Is Your Diet Soda Killing You? on page 107). Post-menopausal women who drank the equivalent of two diet sodas daily were found to be 30 percent more likely to suffer a heart attack or stroke and 50 percent more likely to die from complications of heart disease.

Patients often tell me how they sacrifice with sugar-free diets, and most have happy endings. Living without sugar beverages is life changing for many people, and the improved health benefits can be just as sweet.

YOU MAY BE 1 OF THE 13 MILLION TO BENEFIT FROM THIS NEWS

"All the cardiology residents take statins." No lie. It just rolled off her tongue. A future cardiologist, the fourth-year medical student eagerly shared the underground information. I remember hearing similar stories in the past but had never inquired further.

She went on to explain that (in her experience) residents training as heart specialists had been profoundly aware for years of the benefits of statins, and many young doctors had begun taking the medication as primary prevention against heart disease in order to reap healthy benefits later in life.

Until recently there have been no long-term studies to justify wider use among populations. Now the cat is out of the bag. Widespread use of statins is medically justified and newsworthy. New guidelines accepted by the American Heart Association and the American College of Cardiology will change the way medical providers approach cholesterol management and improve reductions in heart disease.

Instead of trying to achieve aggressively low LDL ("bad cholesterol") levels in all people, the new treatment approach for many patients will focus on the 10-year risk of cardiovascular (heart) disease. The recommendation is to treat those with a risk greater than 7.5 percent of a heart attack, stroke or similar event in the next 10 years.

Let me try my best to hit the latest statin highlights and clarify the significance of this information:

1. 84 percent of men and 53.6 percent of women ages 60-75 years old would be affected by new statin-use guidelines.
2. Approximately 48.6 percent of adults ages 40-75 (56 million people) could be eligible to receive statin therapy.
3. The new guidelines estimate that 14.4 million adults would be eligible to receive statin therapy.
4. Approximately 1.6 million adults previously eligible based on older statin guidelines could discontinue their medication.
5. Statin intervention could result in large cost-savings in quality and quantity of life.

In my clinic, I simplify a patient's risk calculation with a Cardiovascular Risk Assist app. You may try this at home. Here is all you need to know to estimate your 10-year risk for heart disease:

1. Demographics. The calculation is inclusive for African American and non-Hispanic white men and women ages 40-79.*
2. Cholesterol (both total and LDL cholesterol)
3. Systolic blood pressure (top number of your blood pressure reading)
4. Medical information: any current history of high blood pressure, diabetes or smoking

Once you have your risk assessment, the abundance of information may create consumer confusion. Believe me, it is also clinically disruptive. Change is difficult for a doctor as much as it is for patients. ☛

---

*Cardiac risk calculations may underestimate heart disease risks in American Indians, Hispanics and some groups of south Asian ancestry (e.g., Philippines). The calculations may overestimate risks for other populations such as people of east Asian ancestry and Mexican Americans.

SPICE IT UP AND ADD YEARS TO YOUR LIFE

My husband says something so painful must be good for you, and I agree. When treating patients with cold and flu symptoms, I advise a drive over to my favorite Thai restaurant, Thai Thumbz, for a delicious bowl of tom kha soup. The chicken broth has a favorable effect on respiratory illness recovery and the spicy flavors will clear any stuffy nose. That's good news if you have a cold. Now I have even better news. Recent evidence suggests that spicy food is associated with a reduced risk for death.

A recent BMJ journal released a study suggesting that eating spicy foods once or twice weekly could reduce overall death by up to 10 percent. For daily hard-core consumers of spices, the risk of overall death may be reduced to 14 percent.

Researchers report that spicy-food eaters had lower levels of heart and lung disease with reduced cancer rates. Both fresh and dried chili peppers were the most common spices consumed by study participants. Capsaicin was the most common ingredient in the tested spices. A key ingredient found in chili peppers, capsaicin has previously proven to be a beneficial antioxidant with anti-inflammatory effects. It is a chemical that produces a sensation of burning when in contact with mucous membranes such as the mouth and tongue. No pain, no gain!

How hot is really hot? The heat level of chili peppers is measured by Scoville Heat Units (SHU). Higher concentrations of capsaicin result in higher SHU. A bell pepper has 0 units versus a hatch chili, which has 1,000-2,500 units. A habanero chili has 200,000-

350,000 units. Pure capsaicin has—warning, don't try this at home—15,000,000 units.

As far as Thai food, you may want to take this doctor's advice: Use caution when ordering any Thai food spicier than "medium" intensity because the fiery heat will have you sweating bullets. Last time I checked, there was no cure for that ailment. For a gentler culinary experience, enjoy the Hatch Chile Fest at Central Market each August. For healthier living, add some spice to your life! ☛

UNUSUAL MEDICAL BILLING CODES

Y92.241
HURT AT THE LIBRARY

Dr. Sadler brought large marshmallows to the medical school library left over from a school cookout at her ranch. Before she knew it, there were marshmallow wars in the library.

No one was hurt. Two years later she received a package in the mail from the librarian. It was a leftover, withered-up marshmallow found between bookshelves.

PARENTING DOES NOT HAVE TO BE A TRAUMATIC EXPERIENCE

My mother called it "selective amnesia." It was not until the birth of her fifth child (delivered within eight years of the first), that she and my father elected to stop having more babies. In a dual-working-parent household, life was rather chaotic. At one point, all the kids were involved in at least three extracurricular activities, and the family station wagon showed the wear and tear. The large metallic wagon—Mrs. Beasley, we called it—managed to make it through our elementary years and withstand most of our college years.

Although Mrs. Beasley deserves some recognition, credit belongs to my parents, who somehow successfully raised all five of us to become doctors or lawyers.

Mom insists she remembers only the best of our childhood experiences. I do not believe her, but I will keep her secret.

According to the journal Demography (2015), statistically my parents might have stopped after their first child, whose relentless colic and "terrible 2s" were challenging. Nevertheless, they persisted in having more munchkins.

In this scientific article, researchers evaluated parental well-being following the birth of their first child. Using positive and negative parental experiences as predictors of having a second child, they found that a parent's experience with the first birth was a determining factor when it came to deciding family size. According to researchers, the transition into parenthood may be more difficult than expected and many couples choose to have only one child. A young couple in my office today was further testimony to this trend. "This is it!" they announced as their wobbly toddler ran head first into the exam table.

The *Washington Post* reported that having children could be "devastatingly bad." Their sources equate the adverse events associated with parenting as equivalent to or worse than unemployment, divorce or the death of a partner.

Approximately 30 percent of 2,016 German women studied remained at the same level of happiness or better since the birth of their first baby; sadly, however, the majority of women reported decreased happiness the first and second years after giving birth.

Personalizing both my own and my mother's experience with infantile colic and the terrible 2s, it is not difficult to remember all the great parenting experiences and forget the tantrums and dirty diapers. It is like watching your own Facebook account, where you post only happy pictures and positive comments to read like a fairy tale story.

Thank goodness my parents were persistent and hopeful and my sister's symptoms eventually improved. Perhaps as suggested via the American Psychological Association, it is the memories we choose to maintain and the positive experiences we retain that affect our decision- making, particularly when it comes to expanding our own families.

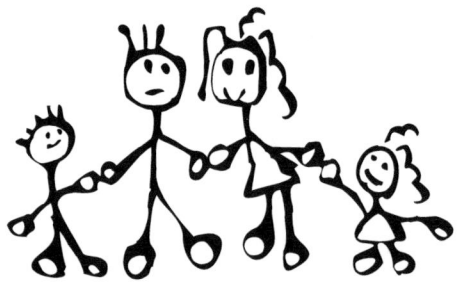

7 REFRIGERATOR-WORTHY HEALTHY HABITS TO MAINTAIN YOUR STUDENT'S HEALTH

Get out your magnets and get ready to post another item on your already crowded refrigerator. You have enough on your plate (and your refrigerator), so I will keep it simple.

How our kids perform in school is important to all parents. If I could narrow down a few home responsibilities and actions that could positively impact academic outcomes, then perhaps this blog is worth your precious parenting time and refrigerator space. The school year has just begun, and just like your New Year's resolutions it is time to remind ourselves and our kids how to stay healthy:

1. Eat the breakfast of champions. Do not let kids skip breakfast. I am surprised by the number of little patients who go without breakfast. Even a breakfast drink is better than nothing and can improve your child's school behavior and grades.

2. The standard brown lunch bag should look like a rainbow inside! Food should be colorful. Red and purple fruits and vegetables contain high levels of anthocyanins, which may reduce the risk of some cancers, heart disease and stroke. Avoid serving or buying foods that are white or yellow, such as fried foods or foods high in carbohydrates.

3. The sound of silence is best when the lights go out at night. A healthier night's sleep is guaranteed when electronics are off and noise eliminated. Remove those headphones from your slumbering child.

4. Keep up with sleep because you cannot catch up. A Harvard study found that even 10 hours of sleep catch-up does not compensate for two weeks of 6-hour nightly sleep. Reaction times of these sleep-deprived individuals were similar to that of people who had pulled all-nighters. Try to have your kids sleep 8-10 hours every night.

5. Healthy teeth, healthy life. While there is no evidence that gum disease is directly linked to heart disease, infected and inflamed gums could indicate self-neglect and are commonly associated with other chronic diseases (diabetes and heart disease). Emphasis on good dental health can improve your child's self-esteem and reduce their dental visits and health care costs.

6. Lighten your load. Does your child really need all that weight in his/her purse or backpack? Better yet (if possible), remove unnecessary items all together. I used to carry a heavy chemistry book "just in case" I needed it. Turned out, I never needed the book and its extra 5 pounds! One study found that student backpacks averaged 18.4 pounds, but some weighed 30 pounds. The American Academy of Pediatrics recommends that backpacks weigh no more than 10-20 percent of the child's body weight. Periodically weigh your child and his/her backpack.

7. Flu shots for everyone! Keep your child in school and away from the sick clinic. In Central Texas, there were a reported 2.4 million school absences, accounting for $91 million in lost revenue to local school districts. The 2014 data attributed half of these events to the flu. While a flu shot is not 100 percent effective (as we learned last year), it is protective, and immunization benefits far outweigh any risks from the vaccine.

If this information meets refrigerator standards, pin it up. Good luck and enjoy a healthy year! ☛

HAND SANITIZING: SKIP THE SCRUB AND GO FOR THE SQUIRT?

Scrub up! It is school time and germs are flying. To be honest, germs generally do not fly. While some may go airborne, most germs rest in your nose and mouth and, with good hygiene, you can keep most of them to yourself.

It is our hands that generally serve as vectors (transport vehicles) for our germs.

Getting rid of bad germs requires repetitive cleaning remedies. In a busy classroom setting, most children will rush through the tedious sanitizing ritual of lathering up and rinsing off. It is much easier to gather a dollop of hand sanitizer than to spend extra time washing with soap and water. So why not skip the scrub and go for the squirt? The Public Library of Science (2014) found that placing hand sanitizers within the classroom made no difference in the numbers of school children's illnesses or absences.

Nonetheless, getting kids to wash with both soap and water can be grueling. As a parent observer and previous classroom volunteer, assisting loads of kids with hand washing is like being part of a pit crew at the Indy 500 car race.

In hospitals, however, use of hand sanitizers has been shown to reduce hospital-based infections. I am sure the easier accessibility of hand cleansers and the greater attention to hand hygiene and infection control must be given much credit for successful reductions in the spread of disease within hospitals.

The Centers for Disease Control and Prevention (CDC) emphasizes that washing hands with soap and water is the best way to reduce bacteria. Alcohol-based hand sanitizers are a reasonable option when access to suds is not available. However, an effective hand sanitizer is one that contains at least 60 percent alcohol, so read labels because not all hand sanitizers are created equal. Hand sanitizers also may not work well if hands are dirty and greasy. Be sure to use the hand sanitizer between the fingers and over the top of the hands as well as on your palms.

As for soap and water, any soap is fine, according to a 2007 University of Michigan study. Here are the five steps to cleaning hands:

1. Wet
2. Lather
3. Scrub for at least 20 seconds, about the time it takes to sing Happy Birthday
4. Rinse (warm or cool water, it does not matter)
5. Dry (with a clean cloth or air dry).

Think that is difficult? In health care settings, medical providers with the World Health Organization scrub for a minimum of 40-60 seconds, and there are 10 steps instead of five!

An interesting caveat: My child's science project discovered the highest germ counts on top of the hand sanitizer dispenser! I suppose the news should be reassuring because we know their dirty hands are getting the squirt. ☛

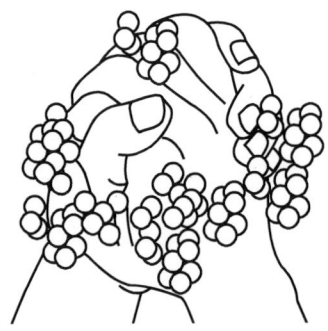

4 NONFICTION FACTS FOR 4 FLU FOLKTALES

I apologize for writing so much on the flu vaccine and its significance in preventing disease and death. As a busy practicing physician, the unintended consequences of bypassing this valuable and affordable vaccine can be devastating.

Fewer than half the people in the United States receive the annual flu vaccine. In my practice I find that there are many reasons people choose to avoid the flu vaccine, and I must put aside my personal opinion and adhere to their wishes. There are repetitive anti-flu themes that arise in conversation with some patients, and I have sectioned their concerns into four groups:

1. People who decline the shot because they believe it is "too early in the season" or it is "too late" in the season.
2. People who claim they get sick after the flu shot.
3. People who claim they never had the flu until they had the flu shot.
4. People who "never had the flu and don't need the shot." Here is how I reply to each group:

Group 1. Flu season is from October to May. The flu vaccine may take up to two weeks for the body to develop antibodies. September is NOT too early, and the Centers for Disease Control and Prevention (CDC) recommends that flu vaccine continues to be offered throughout the flu season, even into March.

Group 2. A randomized control trial demonstrated no difference in side-effect outcomes from the flu shot versus a placebo shot (containing no medicine). The only difference was redness at the injection site and muscle soreness at the injection site (CDC).

Group 3. The flu shot cannot give you the flu, whether you receive a killed virus (in the injectable form) or the attenuated live virus (FluMist). On rare occasions, some of my patients report a low-grade fever and general muscle aches, but these symptoms generally resolve in 1-2 days and are NOT the flu.

Group 4. Why get the flu shot if you have never had the flu? Because you love your friends, kids and parents! The flu shot saves lives and reduces hospitalizations in both pediatric and adult populations. One study demonstrated that an increase in flu vaccination numbers resulted in a decline in flu-related hospitalizations among adults during the 2011-2012 flu seasons (CDC). The more flu shots delivered in a community, the less regional flu and flu complications such as pneumonia, heart attack and death.

More questions about the flu vaccine effectiveness and safety? Please visit the highly informative CDC website, cdc.gov, for more information, plus review all concerns with your medical provider. ☛

> Did you know?: We are still seeing influenza (flu)! If you develop fever, body aches, sore throat and cough, see your medical provider within 24-48 hours of symptoms. With early diagnosis, treatment can lessen the duration and severity of symptoms.

SHRINK ABOUT IT: PRESCRIPTION ESTROGEN WITH DIABETES

Save the brain! An important news release from the American Academy of Neurology caught my eye the other day. Shrinking brain tissue in menopause sounds like a hot topic and certainly this news is highly attention-grabbing, especially for my postmenopausal patients who seek hormone therapy.

A recent analysis demonstrates that type 2 diabetic women on estrogen therapy had decreased brain volume compared to their non-estrogen-treated diabetic and non-diabetic counterparts. Women in the trial were at least 65 years of age, and some were placed on placebo (sugar pills) or 0.625 mg of estrogen with or without progesterone. There were approximately 1,400 participants, so this was not a small study and neither was the volume of brain shrinkage.

In the study's first 30 months, the diabetic women on estrogen therapy had an average 18 milliliters less total brain volume in gray matter compared to their female diabetic and non-diabetic counterparts.

I am oversimplifying this information (the neurologists must be rolling their eyes). The brain is composed primarily of two tissue types: white matter and gray matter. White matter serves primarily to cable information between both sides of the brain and regulate unconscious functions such as body temperature, respiration and heart rate. Gray matter is responsible for memory, attention, consciousness and thoughts. Loss of gray matter in the brain is commonly found in people with Alzheimer's disease, a common form of dementia.

In a review article, Dr. Hugenshmidt of Wake Forest University suggests that estrogen interferes with glucose metabolism in the brain and may lead to decreased brain gray matter (brain tissue). Diabetics have abnormal glucose metabolism, and estrogen may amplify these adverse effects in the brain's gray matter. Another recent study linked decreased brain glucose metabolism to worsening memory function.

At the end of 30 months, the study found that despite the loss of significant gray matter volume, there were no significant differences in cognitive scores according to the Mini Mental Status Exam.* I am sure that repeat testing is planned and the results will impact decision-making for patients and doctors on whether to continue hormone replacement therapy whether or not diabetes exists. My philosophy on hormone replacement has always been "the lowest dose for the shortest amount of time," and this study confirms that.

Save your brain. If you are diabetic and on hormone therapy, be sure to review the risks and benefits of continued treatment. I hope this provides you more information to shrink about! ☞

*The Mini Mental Status Exam measures appearance, language, cognitive skills, orientation, memory and judgment skills.

A double-wide tale! When Dr. Jane's family first acquired the family farm, they slept on cots and used the old wooden outhouse. The outhouse was a "double-wide" 2-seater customized for both children and adults.

SKIP THE SUPPLEMENT: FISH ARE FRIENDS AND FOOD

I loved the movie *Finding Nemo*. My first pet was "Fighty," a betta fish. A mirror strategically placed in front of his aquarium produced an image he saw as competitive, causing him to puff out his gills and show off his colorful fins. Fighty was great for developing my (much) younger growing mind, and caring for him taught me responsibility. Above all, he was my friend.

As a grown-up, I still love fish—but now, grilled or baked. I know. A terrible blog intro, but perhaps I have your attention.

Fish is considered a brain-healthy food with high levels of omega-3 fatty acids, which can help slow memory loss and even help prevent Alzheimer's disease. Other beneficial brain foods include walnuts, eggs, spinach and blueberries. Green leafy vegetables contain lutein and zeaxanthin, which may slow mental decline by as much as 40 percent.

Fresh foods, however, require refrigeration and frequent grocery shopping. Vitamins and other nutritional supplements therefore seem easier to obtain, have longer shelf lives and claim to have highly concentrated nutrients. BUT NOT SO FAST...

The Journal of the American Medical Association (August 2015) discovered that older adults who took nutritional supplements with omega-3 fatty acids and a combination of lutein and zeaxanthine experienced the same level of intellectual decline over a five-year period as those who took placebo pills.

In other words, eat your greens and enjoy fish high in omega-3 fatty acids. Diets such as the DASH diet and the Mediterranean diet are notably good for both the heart and the mind.

For the record, I would never have eaten my betta fish; he died of natural causes. ☛

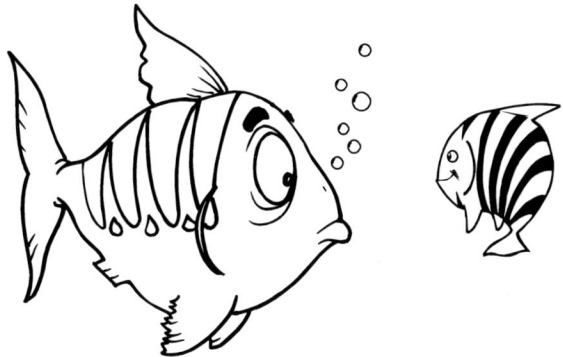

5 MYTHS AND 5 RECOVERY TOOLS FOR CELEBRATING THE NEW YEAR

I will be out of the clinic Jan. 1, so let me make it clear that if you are my patient and are looking to recover from your celebratory New Year's event, I will be unavailable. That said, here is some free advice for all of you that may or may not be useful (you will see what I mean).

A hangover may be caused by a combination of the toxic effects of excessive alcohol to the brain, physiologic response to withdrawal,* and the metabolic breakdown of alcohol's chemicals. Symptoms include headache, fatigue, nausea, dizziness, sensitivity to sight and sound, and rapid heartbeat. A hangover depends on how much a person drinks and the type (concentration) of alcohol consumed. Symptoms begin as blood alcohol levels drop and may last up to 24 hours.

When I read that a clinic in Australia specializes in hangover recovery, I thought I'd better inform people of the simple truth: Treatment following "a belly full of booze" is just "boogering around" (i.e., wasting your time). *Look it up, my Aussie wordage is correct!* At a cost of up to $200 per hour, intravenous fluids, vitamins and oxygen therapy will do nothing but empty your wallet.

As a family practice physician, I am the queen of preventative care. The best treatment remedy for a hangover is *avoiding excessive alcohol*. Hold on! Before you call me a party pooper, let me explain why my reasoning is absolutely correct.

True or false:

1. Many people believe they are immune to hangovers. **False.** According to researchers with the European College of Neuropsychopharmacology, there is a direct relationship between how much alcohol is consumed and the risk for hangover. Simple math.

2. Eating a heavy meal following alcohol consumption reduces hangover symptoms. **False.** Rumor (and literary searches) have it that students will try consuming a heavy, fat-laden meal after excessive alcohol consumption. Not helpful, according to the study.

3. Drinking plenty of fluids before or during an alcohol binge reduces hangover symptoms. **False.** While there may be some truth that people who alternate water or hydrating solutions in-between alcoholic beverages may drink overall less alcohol, fluid hydration does not prevent or reduce the headache, nausea and fatigue associated with post-party binges.

4. Taking acetaminophen (e.g., Tylenol) before bedtime makes the morning after a little easier. **False.** Acetaminophen is metabolized through the liver and compounds the potential toxic effects of alcohol on the liver. Ibuprofen may be a better choice for post-holiday headaches.

5. Treating alcohol hangover with more alcohol. **False.** It is adding fuel to the fire. Do not do it.

What does work:

1. Drinking fluids in-between alcoholic drinks will fill you up and you might drink less.
2. Drinking in moderation. In other words, limit yourself to fewer than two regular-size drinks. One drink is defined as 12 ounces of beer, 5 ounces of wine or 1½ ounces of 80-proof liquor.

3. Fruit juice or sports drinks (Gatorade or Powerade) might be helpful for recovery. In addition, clear broth soups may be helpful. These electrolyte-rehydration solutions could be helpful.

4. Plan a day of rest following heavy alcohol intake. Do not attempt to perform complex tasks the day after a substantial drinking binge. A person's degree of precision performance is generally hampered due to lingering alcohol effects.

5. If you must choose medication for symptom relief, consider ibuprofen for headaches. Add an antacid or proton-pump inhibitor (e.g., Prilosec). Alcohol can cause temporary inflammation to the stomach lining, which can be made worse with ibuprofen. Keep your bases covered.

Good luck with your post-celebratory symptoms. Be sure to have a designated driver if you plan to drink and travel to your party. Remember, the best medicine is preventative medicine (coming from this family doctor), and my best advice remains the same: Limit alcohol intake and you will find that Jan. 1, 2016, is far more enjoyable! ☞

*Alcohol being removed from the body is suspected to be a contributory cause to hangover symptoms. These symptoms are separate and NOT related to alcohol addiction and withdrawal.

ARE STETHOSCOPES GOING THE WAY OF THE TYPEWRITER, OR JUST AGING GRACEFULLY?

Sitting at a heart-sound conference several years ago, I spent hours listening to the multitude of heart murmurs and memorizing and correlating heart sounds with physical heart abnormalities. My mother, a family doctor, sat next to me and the two of us trained our ears to better interpret the gentle "swish" or "whoosh" of the sounds within the heart rhythm to connect the murmurs to physical heart abnormalities. Probably one of my more difficult medical meetings, because at times listening to the similarity of sounds was admittedly agonizing.

Then today I read "The stethoscope is dead." and "The time for the stethoscope is gone." *What is that all about?* Reading on, another physician replied, "We are not at the place, and probably won't be for a very long time...it is valuable." OK, I can take another breath (and I will use my stethoscope to hear it)!

The stethoscope spat has been around for a while. Studies have shown that cardiology fellows (trainees) will diagnose murmurs accurately up to 56 percent of the time and internal medicine residents about 36 percent of the time. With repetition and repeated auscultatory training, diagnostic capabilities improved. However, neither physician group improved any more than the auditory skills of third-year medical students. The ease of technology and ultrasound (echocardiogram) accuracy has led to more rapid diagnostic techniques that are far better than most trained ears. I know a cardiologist who tells me, "When I hear a murmur, I just slap the ultrasound on their chest," so she can more accurately determine its cause.

Used in most office visits, my stethoscope is an important tool to screen for heart abnormalities. It aids in detecting pneumonias, asthma complications, blood vessel weaknesses (aneurysms) and so much more. Heck, I even use it for a reflex hammer! When I don't wear a white coat, it is my uniform. In fact, for TV interviews I am always asked to wear it. My stethoscopes even come in stylish colors. OK, I have said enough. For now, I am keeping my stethoscope. Just like me (I hope), I will let it age gracefully. ☛

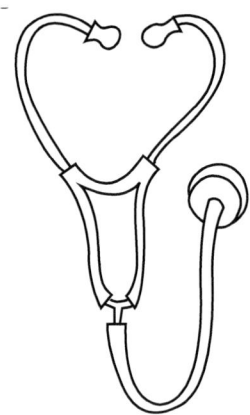

DOES A FULL MOON AFFECT YOUR MOOD? TRUTH BE TOLD...

"It is going to be a busy night. Full moon!" barked my chief resident. Heeding his warning, we seemed more prepared and less surprised by the large influx of sick people entering the emergency department. The residency culture surrounding high-patient-volume nights with a full moon continues today. This misguided folklore has been passed on to generations of interns.

Several years ago (1987), a study revealed that 80 percent of nurses and up to 64 percent of emergency room doctors believed there was a significant lunar affect on patients. Of the nurses polled, 92 percent suggested a "differential pay schedule" for these particularly more stressful night shifts.

The Roman goddess of the moon is Luna, and lunar comes from the Latin word *luna*, meaning the moon. *Luna* is also the prefix of the word "lunatic" and is associated with an old belief that the moonlight made people mad; for centuries, people have believed that the lunar cycle has an effect on mood.

Attention shoppers! Time to bring you all up to date. The full moon is not associated with increased numbers of patients seeking urgent medical treatment for psychological anxiety, and the lunar cycle has no impact on the number of cases in emergency rooms.

Hang on, there is more to the story (based on facts). A recent study confirms that the moon's cycle *does* influence sleep. Current Biology (2013) studied group participants' sleep-time brain waves (electroencephalogram) and blood melatonin levels. In addition, the study followed both sleep duration and quality. Researches discovered a lunar rhythm.

Here is what can happen during a full moon:

1. Total sleep time was reduced by 20 minutes. Prepare ahead of time, aim for earlier sleep or choose to pattern your sleep with the moon. However, decreased duration of sleep is associated with depression and obesity. Every minute counts!

2. The quality and length of deep sleep decreased by 30 percent. Deep sleep is important because that is when the body repairs and rebuilds tissues and strengthens bones and the immune system.

3. Time to fall asleep increased by five minutes. EVERY MINUTE OF SLEEP COUNTS.

4. Subjective sleep quality decreased. People did not feel they experienced the same quality of sleep during full-moon nights. These subjects did not even know there was a full moon. Very interesting. It is possible that humans follow the lunar cycle in their sleep habits, and this could account for changes in sleep quality.

5. Blood melatonin levels decreased during a full moon. Melatonin is an important hormone released from the pineal gland in the brain and helps regulate our internal body clock. Melatonin is at its highest in the evening and is important because it controls the release of some female reproductive hormones and may help to regulate the menstrual cycle. Low levels of melatonin may be related to aging, as lower levels are seen in older adults

You may not go mad during a full moon, but it is best you prepare to get better sleep. Exercise, drink plenty of fluids during the day, and arrive to bed a bit earlier than usual. You may feel a little better on those days following a full moon.

GOT PERIMENOPAUSE? STIMULATE YOUR SKIN TO KEEP IT SMOOTHER

Mirror mirror on the wall
My skin was like a china doll's.
But perimenopause does call
Now my skin now just wants to fall.

It sags, it wrinkles through my ages
But time cannot be kept in cages.
The creams, the rubs and lathered greases
Will never keep away deep creases.

Mirror mirror on the wall
I'll love my wrinkles after all!
(Now made clear for you to see
My gift is not my poetry.)

    Hot flashes, irregular periods, hair loss and other midlife perimenopause symptoms can adversely affect quality of life. After an escalation of symptoms, full-blown menopause strikes. For many, the entire experience is like a gentle breeze. For other women, menopause can be uncomfortable, prolonged and far less simple. Increasingly, information is pointing in the direction of aggressively managing estrogen support during a window around menopause. A bridge of estrogen therapy may promote improved bone health, help relieve hot flashes and (yes!) improve skin tone. During this time, evidence is beginning to emerge supporting both estrogen therapy and collagen simultaneously as a method to preserve skin matrix and promote collagen building.

The American Academy of Dermatology's summer 2015 meeting disclosed studies supporting a "timing hypothesis" of estrogen use that could help decrease collagen loss in perimenopausal women. According to the report, some types of collagen decrease by up to 50 percent within a few years of menopause. This loss of collagen is related directly to the loss of estrogen within the skin's matrix. Within the skin, estrogen receptors bind to estrogen and help to promote collagen building. These estrogen receptors decline as we age. However, the timing hypothesis suggests that added estrogen provided to these skin receptors during this window of opportunity could optimize collagen formation.

During this perimenopausal time, the skin seems primed for collagen stimulation with physical or chemical treatments. The dermatologists suggest laser resurfacing, microneedling (i.e., SkinPen) or radiofrequency, among other available treatments. In other words: Go after the collagen while it is still present and primed for rejuvenation and the estrogen receptors are up and running! ☛

DON'T BURY YOUR HEAD IN THE SAND; ENJOY THE BEACH

Beach season is upon us, and it is time to pack your first aid kit before heading to the shoreline. What do you fear most at the beach? Many people would say sharks. As a well-traveled Texan with medical experience, I would be more concerned about hitting a deer on the highway, getting bit by a dog in the parking lot or being knocked over by a roving cow.

Once you hit the beach, anticipating common seaside injuries may help you avoid seeking professional medical attention. Here is a list of five most common shoreline injuries and their treatment:

1. Sunburn affects up to 30 percent of adults and up to 70 percent of children and adolescents every year. Prevention is most important, and applying sunscreen with SPF of 30 or greater is recommended. Reapply it every two to three hours and as soon as you dry off after coming out of the water. If you experience discomfort from a mild sunburn, an aloe-based cream or topical lidocaine (Dermoplast) can be helpful. For more painful and severe sunburns, it may be best to seek medical advice.

2. Jellyfish stings affect up to 150 million people annually; up to 200,000 jellyfish injuries occur in Florida alone. Common signs and symptoms of jellyfish stings include a rash and burning, prickling and stinging sensations. The Portuguese man-of-war and bluebottle jellyfish are common to the Florida coast. Multiple stings or certain highly toxic jellyfish exposures may cause nausea, vomiting, headache and fever.

Vinegar, a hot-water rinse (115 degrees F) or a paste made of baking soda work best to denature the venom. To remove attached stingers, use tweezers and a magnifying glass. Care must be taken not to open the venomous sack attached to some of these stingers. Specialists recommend scraping the stingers off with a blunt tool such as a tongue-blade or the edge of a credit card. Oral antihistamines such as diphenhydramine and skin steroid creams (cortisone) can ease the discomfort. Despite what you have heard, urinating on the jellyfish sting is not a recommended remedy.

To minimize toxic jellyfish exposure, wear a protective suit when in the water. Some stores sell protective "stinger suits" made of thin, high-tech fabric.

3. Beach glass and sharp rocks can cause superficial scrapes or deep skin cuts. Carry along your standard first aid kit and check your antibiotic creams to make certain they are not expired. Keep ice-bag packets in the cooler to ease pain and decrease swelling. Waterproof bandages can be found at your local pharmacy. Tetanus immunizations should be renewed every 10 years.

4. Sea "lice," fire coral and sea urchin exposure can cause significant rash, sometimes with a prickly sensation. With sea lice, the "sea bather's itch" may occur a few hours to days after exposure to ocean water. Sea lice derives from contact with the infantile form (larvae) of the thimble jellyfish. Fire coral (not coral) is a cousin to the jellyfish, looks like seaweed and has stingers. Very intense itching and redness is the hallmark of this rash. Aveeno oatmeal baths, cortisone over the counter, diphenhydramine, and acetaminophen or ibuprofen can be helpful. If the rash worsens, see your medical provider or, like my British and Egyptian cousins, lift up your shirt in the middle of a restaurant to ask your physician family member the source and treatment of your rash! If you plan to swim in ocean waters, wear protective clothing and remove swimsuits immediately after use (of course, put something else on!). Rinse garments in warm water and detergent daily.

5. Watch for shark advisories and be cautious when swimming in shark-friendly waters (such as near large, dead carcasses). My medical advice for shark bites: Get out of the water as soon as possible, stop the bleeding and call 911. The good news is that there are only 65 shark attacks worldwide each year, and only a small number are fatal. You are three times more likely to drown at the beach and 30 times more likely to be killed by lightning than to die from a shark attack, according to the University of Florida's International Shark Attack File. So, as I mentioned before...on your way to the beach, watch out for deer, dogs and cows. ☛

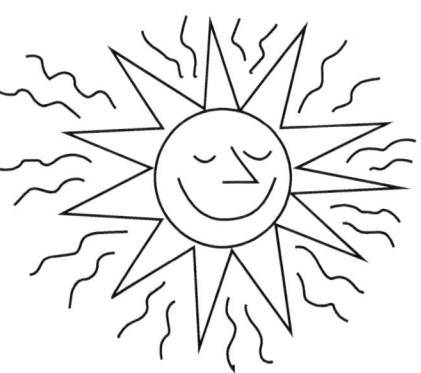

CALORIES DON'T COUNT WHEN I STEAL THEM OFF YOUR PLATE

I never order my own French fries. Instead, I sneak the crispy critters off the family's dinner plates. In my mind, this choice method deletes the food off my calorie rap sheet. My family puts up with my habit because they have no choice. In anticipation of maternal fry-loss, my son requests an additional side order at In-N-Out Burger. To me, food tastes better off someone else's plate and has far fewer calories. But who's counting?

Scientists challenged the calorie-counting weight-loss methods by contesting that "a calorie is not a calorie." In October 2014, authors Sean Lucan and James DiNicolantonia (Public Health Nutrition) placed greater emphasis on higher quality whole foods instead of high sugars and starchy processed "lower quality" foods. Even when the calorie content is similar, the physiologic effects on body weight and body fat can be very different.

An example compared a calorie's worth of high-protein salmon and healthy olive oil versus a calorie's worth of a simple carbohydrate such as white rice. These foods affect hormones in different ways and may positively or negatively impact our hunger, weight control, food consumption and body composition.

The New England Journal of Medicine in 2011 found foods such as vegetables, nuts, fruits and whole grains were associated with less weight gain. In addition, high-fiber foods augmented satiety. Yogurt consumption was associated with less weight gain. On the other hand, overall changes in consumption of all liquids except milk were associated with more weight gain. Researchers found high associations of weight gain with consumption of starches, refined grains and processed foods. Scientists hypothesized that these starchy foods are less satiating and increase hunger (hormone) signals compared to higher fiber foods that contain equivalent calories but contain healthy fats and proteins (such as olive oil and salmon).

My mother and sister used to count calories incessantly. Our kitchen was adorned with small scraps of paper covered with calorie counts. To me, it was too much trouble. I never counted calories. Perhaps I was better off. Perhaps not all calories are the same and we should focus on what kind of food we eat and not solely rely on caloric content. If we control total calorie intake and account for exercise calories burned, there are qualitative differences in calories consumed. ☞

> Matt Damon, actor and co-founder of water.org, has said he will "not be going to the bathroom" until there is clean sanitation for everyone. Well, he is NOT the Bust of the Week (although his efforts are admirable)—that honor goes to the morning newscaster who said you cannot die from not going to the bathroom.
>
> Yes, you can die if you completely stop urinating or defecating. A good example is people who suffer urinary obstruction. They are at risk for a deadly infection of the kidneys and blood and can be at risk for kidney or other organ failure. In addition, inability to have a bowel movement can result in bowel obstruction and perforation (a tear) of the colon, which is another deadly case scenario. Careful, careful! You are the same newscaster who blamed your co-anchor's flu on a flu shot (false!). Leave the medical advice to the experts!

MY COLD HAS GONE VIRAL!

Runny nose, low-grade fever, cough and fatigue. My symptoms began yesterday and have escalated to a full-blown cold. Like many people, I will push through and manage the symptoms at home. Like I tell my patients, it has only been a few days and there is no reason to seek medical attention. Most colds are viral, and prompt recovery does not necessitate an antibiotic prescription.

According to the Annals of Internal Medicine (January 2016), more than 90 percent of people with similar symptoms as mine have a viral illness. Although I feel ill, and I am contagious, an antibiotic will not decrease my level of contagiousness, could hinder my recovery and may lead to other physical complications.

Before I move on, here is a quiz:

What causes more than 2 million illnesses a year?

What is responsible for more than 23,000 deaths a year?

What costs the U.S. economy more than $30 billion dollars a year?

Answer: Antibiotic resistance, the result of years of repeatedly over-prescribing antibiotics.

An estimated 5-25 percent of patients will experience side effects from their antibiotics, and these prescriptions are responsible for one in every five medication-related emergency room visits. Antibiotic complications include (among others): rash, nausea, vomiting, diarrhea, breathing difficulties and sudden death.

Clostridium difficile, an antibiotic-associated diarrhea, will occur in one of every

1,000 people prescribed these medications. This past year, I have treated two or three seriously ill patients stricken with this ailment. That is testimony to the careful practice and decision-making physicians must use in prescribing antibiotics.

I have only been sick for a few days. But if my symptoms continue for up to 10 days or I develop fever, vomiting, headache or rash, then this doctor will be checking in with her doctor. ☛

She's not pulling your leg...
When Dr. Jane's husband was first introduced to her family, he was quickly greeted, then told to get into the field and assist a birthing cow. Without hesitation, the city boy tied a rope around the calf's legs and with all his own muscle power (and the help of a tractor) he successfully delivered the newborn. Both the calf and John recovered well and John was immediately accepted into the family.

WHAT TO DO WHEN YOU HAVE THE STOMACH FLU

"I really need to clean Samantha's dusty robe!" That is what I believed would be my dying thought as I lay sick on the cold tiles of my daughter's bathroom floor, felled by a stomach bug.

Trying to avoid awakening my husband, I had dragged myself upstairs to my college daughter's empty room.

#doctorscannotbesick messaged one patient when she discovered I was out of the office. I wish. It was a miserable experience and, as I found out, I had PLENTY of company. Several of my friends had also become ill over the weekend, and we had similar gut-wrenching (pardon the pun) stories to share.

Before it strikes your house, you might want to know what you're up against—and how to treat the problem.

Stomach flu, or gastroenteritis, is most commonly a viral infection and less often bacterial or parasitic. It can be spread by food, by direct person-to-person contact or through contact with contaminated surfaces. Rapidly spread, these infections are common among people housed in close quarters.

The Centers for Disease Control and Prevention (CDC) reports norovirus as the most common cause for gastroenteritis among U.S. children, and it is responsible for between 50 and 70 percent of cases in adults. In most cases, diarrhea lasts for five to seven days and vomiting fewer than two days.

Approximately 20 percent of gastroenteritis is due to bacteria such as Salmonella, shigella and E. coli. Hallmark symptoms may include prolonged (more than seven days) symptoms and bloody diarrhea. According to the CDC, the deadliest form of gastroenteritis is Clostridium difficile. This antibiotic-associated bacterium is increasingly found in the community and is contagious; newer forms are becoming more aggressive and deadly (see CDC.gov).

Gastroenteritis is responsible for up to 21 million illnesses, 71,000 hospitalizations and 800 deaths annually in the U.S. In patients with healthy immune systems, most cases do not require antibiotics. In many cases, antibiotics could worsen symptoms of diarrhea and stomach pain, and the CDC discourages its use without identification of a specific cause.

Most gastroenteritis cases can be managed in the home. Here are five tips for a more comfortable journey to wellness:

1. Stay home. Presenteeism (opposite of absenteeism) can only spread the virus and result in less productivity for you. It is highly important not to spread your infection among co-workers! Isolate yourself at home until symptoms subside. After toileting, wash your hands for the length of time it takes to finish singing Happy Birthday.

2. Increase your fluid volume. Rehydrating solutions such as low-sugar G2 (Gatorade), Powerade or Pedialyte are top on the list of this doctor's "feel-better fluids." Full of natural electrolytes, coconut water may be helpful for mild fluid losses. Dr. Mark Miller, gastroenterologist at Baylor Scott & White Health and Digestive Health Associates of Texas, suggests CeraLyte rehydration for patients suffering significant fluid losses. If these methods fail, it is time for intravenous fluid replacement, so head to your local clinic or emergency room.

3. Do not be in a hurry to eat regular food. Wait until the nausea subsides and then

stick with small amounts of bland and salty snacks such as chicken broth and crackers. Advance your diet to more regular foods as your nausea symptoms resolve and your diarrhea lessens. Keep in mind: If it does not seem like it will go down well, then expect the same when it comes back up!

4. Over-the-counter anti-diarrheal and nausea medications may help. If you have severe diarrhea or vomiting, an over-the-counter medication may ease your symptoms. I recommend you contact your medical provider first, as these medications are not recommended for children and for those suffering severe abdominal pain, bloody diarrhea or fever. Prescription medications may also lessen symptoms.

5. Know when to seek medical attention. Contact your medical provider for further advice if you are (or are caring for) a sick elderly or immunocompromised person. In addition, dehydrated infants or young children need more urgent care. For anyone suffering severe abdominal pain, bloody diarrhea, weakness or uncontrolled vomiting and diarrhea, emergent medical evaluation is needed.

For my sweet patient: #DoctorsDOgetsick. For my college daughter: I washed your robe. ☛

> Important "take home message" regarding sunscreen: When it comes to sunscreen, protective active ingredients only last two-three hours (less time if you get in and out of the water). The key to effective sunblock: Reapply, reapply and reapply.

ABOUT THE AUTHOR

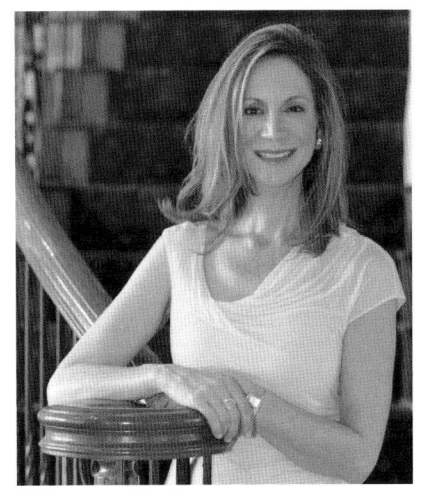

Jane Sadler, M.D.

Shortly after moving to Houston in 1969, my mother announced that our family of six was about to become a family of seven. My father was so surprised that our newly introduced Irish setter nearly fell out of his arms. Luckily, there were four eager daughters ready to gather up the rambunctious puppy. My brother, the "caboose," would be born several months later. Mom began preparing for her return to medicine, we began school, and the house became a real-life zoo.

Dad remained busy in the laboratory, researching treatment strategies for rare endocrine tumors, managing patients and training residents at M.D. Anderson Hospital (now Cancer Center). Over the next 25 years, he contributed to a multitude of research papers and books on hormone-related diseases and cancers. One of the first doctors to successfully manage infertility, my father once received a pair of breeding cattle from a grateful famous rancher. His patients included those with no financial means to those of great wealth and nobility. Never short of fascinating stories, Dad loved to share about the day he found Mr. Packard (of Hewlett-Packard) working underneath his laboratory's malfunctioning radioimmunoassay machine.

I keep a memorable picture of my father, not a man of great height, towering over African pygmies. The African jungle was one of many journeys he took around the world that helped to advance his understanding of growth hormones.

Mom eventually joined a multi-specialty practice. A soft-spoken doctor with a gentle British accent, she was not expected to thrive professionally. On her first day of work, she was provided only a rolling cart with a Rolodex. To her partners' surprise, Mom's practice would quickly flourish and she would become one of the busiest practitioners in her large physician group.

At the peak of her professional career, Mom managed patients in the clinic, taught medical students and cared for patients in several nursing homes and three hospitals (along with looking after five exceptionally busy children). She hired a woman named Faye to help maintain our busy household and drive us to our activities. Faye was a large woman with an even larger heart. Although she did very little housework, spent a lot of time at the kitchen table and loved to watch soap operas, she showed up for work daily. Her reliability earned her tenure (she worked for our family into our adult lives) and a place in our family. Faye's job eventually evolved into post-stroke care when Dad was stricken with tragedy. Faye sat with us at my father's funeral. Not long after his death, we cared for her, honored to sit at her bedside and, later, be present at her funeral.

My mother was Doctor Doolittle. She would insist the parakeets regularly be freed from their cages to fly around the house for exercise. The birds' seeded waste bleached the walls and, like hardened concrete, was impossible to remove. Hoppity, my Dutch rabbit, became a regular Houdini. He would magically disappear from his hutch. After freely roaming the house, Hoppity regularly left a trail of small, round poop. My unfortunate brother—I should not have told him they were chocolate chips. Hoppity was the only bunny to avoid being killed by the dogs, so he grew old and toothless. Not one to let any animal die without her life-saving efforts, Mom regularly hand-fed Hoppity softened oatmeal. Our kitchen was becoming an official pet triage area.

Three litters of Irish setters, countless bunnies, rescued baby blue jays and 10 unintentional chicks (the result of mistakenly leaving a laboratory experiment's incubator on over the weekend) were only a few of the many animals to inhabit our household. After we bought a small weekend family farm outside of Houston, our suburban Houston home would serve as a refuge for baby farm animals and our family station wagon as their transport vehicle.

In our living room, an orphaned calf would rest on our laps; we thought nothing of bottle-feeding her while we sat on the couch. Most memorable was my calf Jeffrey. Barely conscious, uttering occasional baby moos, the helpless newborn calf lay on our bathroom floor. Jeffrey had a feeding tube inserted through his nose into his stomach. His sour milk smell filled the small room but was easily forgiven. He was not to live on the bathroom floor for more than a few days. I came home from school to feed Jeffrey on his third day of life, but he was gone.

My parents purchased horses for us to ride at the ranch. They were not well-trained and neither were we. Mom insisted we learn to ride without saddles, assuring us we would learn to become better riders. After several falls and a broken arm, the saddles arrived. My first and most memorable horse was Scarlett. Neither one of us formally trained, we competed in only one small show alongside several fancy pure-bred horses. We placed fifth in Western pleasure and I still have my trophy; it is one of my greatest triumphs.

In high school I played violin, studied with a violinist from the Houston Symphony and became the high school orchestra concert mistress. I walked away from the violin my senior year to become flag corps captain of the marching band. At the same time, I began teaching aerobics at a local dance studio.

As the youngest student instructor, I quickly learned how to work with adult students and instructors. Jane Fonda had famously hit the video exercise scene, and aerobic dance went viral. Along with other adult instructors, I was invited to meet and work out with the exercise icon, fit in her familiar striped leotard. She was encouraging to our large group. I was in my element, and chose to pursue exercise physiology as my path through college.

I continued to teach and train aerobics instructors into college and medical school. My fellow instructors included Candy, Mitzi, Buffy and Muffy (no kidding). We were occasionally invited to exercise the Texas A&M University football team on post-game Sundays in the esteemed university stadium, Kyle Field.

I credit Dr. Stephen Crouse, previous head of the human performance lab at Texas A&M University (TAMU), with mentoring and encouraging me to pursue medicine. He worked with the school's dean to exchange physical education credits with pre-med requirements. He enabled me to work with the medical school in his human physiology lab to measure performance levels of morning versus evening cortisol levels in the school's cycling team. I gathered some out-of-shape and really good friends for comparison data. Participants celebrated the end of the research at our family farm.

I completed an internship in exercise technology from TAMU on a Friday, graduated on Saturday, had a party on Sunday and began medical school on Monday.

In medical school, I was encouraged to specialize and discouraged from pursuing family medicine, as it was "too generalized." I loved obstetrics and gynecology and chose Parkland Hospital in Dallas (University of Texas Southwestern) for training. It was the most aggressive and challenging residency. At the same time, I had met John, my future husband.

In residency, I loved everything. Surgery was exciting and delivering babies exhilarating, but I really enjoyed the clinical side of women's health along with pediatrics and general medicine. I could do it all with family practice. Changing training programs to family practice is a decision I never regret. I love being my community's doctor.

I am grateful for my encouraging and loving husband, John, who has endured my arduous writing adventures and been my technical help through many speaking engagements. My two wonderful children, Samantha and John Michael, have taught me the complexities of parenting, polished my pediatric skills and loved me unconditionally. I am thankful to Dr. Carl Couch for bringing me to Garland and mentoring me, and being supportive of my career and family. I appreciate Michael Merschel, an editor at the Dallas Morning News, for his continued encouragement in my weekly and monthly publishing, and Susan Hall with Baylor Scott & White public relations, who for years has allowed me many avenues in which to share my medical knowledge. I live and work in Garland, Texas, and am grateful for my neighbors and local community for their trust in my care.

A special thank you goes out to book editor Anita Robison for her effort and skill she so carefully placed into these pages. Her dedication to detail is outstanding. She gracefully led me through the thick waters of unknown publishing territory. To Janet Long, the book's designer: Your creative thinking helped bring the pages to life and your illustrations molded the stories together. You are both admired and appreciated.

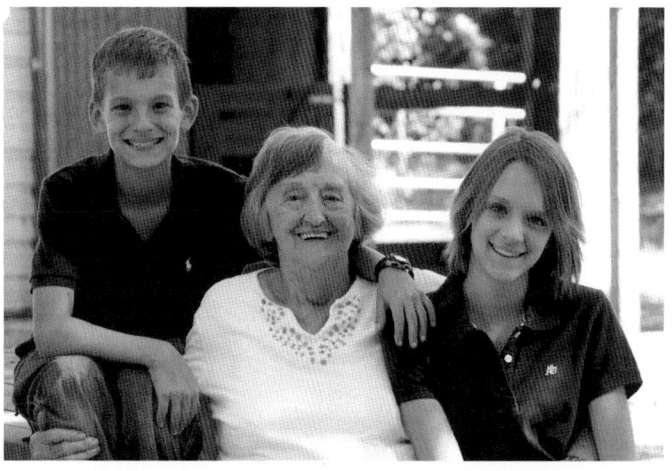

John Michael, Mom and Samantha

One of my favorite Bible passages is from Proverbs 17:22: *A joyful heart is good medicine, but a broken spirit dries up the bones.* Our love for the medical profession can be contagious to both patients and staff. As members of the medical profession, it is important we have joy for our work and those whom we serve.

I credit the culture of my upbringing for how I've turned out. Not in the sense that my father was Egyptian and my mother British, but culture referring to the colorful role we all played as part of a large family full of kids and animals. My working parents served as strong role models and never discouraged me from any activities, no matter how out of place they seemed. My parents embraced change in their own lives by moving across oceans, and their adventures helped shape me into the person I am today.

Read more blogs at www.drjaneexplains.com
Contact her at drjane@drjaneexplains.com
Follow her on Twitter @drjaneexplains